Epidural Technique In Obstetric Anesthesia

Giorgio Capogna

Epidural Technique In Obstetric Anesthesia

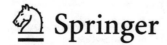 Springer

Giorgio Capogna
European School of Obstetric Anesthesia
Rome
Italy

ISBN 978-3-030-45334-3   ISBN 978-3-030-45332-9   (eBook)
https://doi.org/10.1007/978-3-030-45332-9

This Springer imprint is published by the registered company Springer Nature Switzerland AG
The registered company address is: Gewerbestrasse 11, 6330 Cham, Switzerland

To Rita and Emanuele

Preface

èpi- [from the Greek. ἐπί "above, in, more"]
pèri- [from the Greek. περί, περι- "around"]
èxtra- [from the Latin. extra "outside"]

The terms "epidural," "peridural," and "extradural" are basically synonyms.

To be anatomically precise, peridural should be the most correct term, because it implies that the space is around the dura and therefore it envelops the entire dural sac, while epidural refers to a space that is upon or on the dural sac.

Peridural is most used in countries whose language comes from Latin, extradural is the term currently used in British English-speaking countries, and epidural is currently used in Standard English-speaking countries.

The term "space" is used to indicate the region lying between the dura and the bony walls of the spinal canal. However, the term space is not completely exact, because it is not an empty space, but a place that is filled mainly with fat and with other anatomical structures, and therefore should be called "region" rather than "space." As we will discuss in the chapter devoted to the anatomy, the most recent anatomical findings support the idea that the epidural region is in part real and in part virtual.

In this text, I will use the most commonly used term: epidural space.

Epidural block is a form of peripheral nerve block accomplished by introducing local anesthetic agents into the epidural space. In this way, the local anesthetic affects the nerve fibers beyond their arachnoid-dural coverings as they lie in the intervertebral foramen, paravertebral space, or sacral canal.

Our masters J. J. Bonica and P. Bromage wrote everything that could be said on the subject, for which I will necessarily refer to their teachings; however, more or less 70 years have passed from their cornerstone publications, and some new things have been discovered, some others have been confirmed with modern methods, and new techniques face the horizon. Clinical practice has also slightly changed. For this reason, I wanted to write this book, to transmit their knowledge and experience to the new generations, adding a little of my updated practical experience.

This book is intended for all colleague anesthetists, but in particular those who want to practice or who already practice analgesia in obstetrics, and therefore it will exclusively describe the lumbar approach to the epidural space which is the one used in obstetrics.

The epidural block has been known universally for a long time; however, its specific teaching is beginning to be lost, as this practice is mainly confined within the scope of obstetric analgesia. For this reason, I hope this book will help my young colleagues to learn and appreciate a fundamental technique for the anesthesiologist and my older colleagues to review their technique to better teach it to future generations.

Rome, Italy   Giorgio Capogna

Contents

History of Lumbar Epidural Block

Whether Corning in 1884 had obtained true spinal anesthesia in his first human experiment or had merely produced an epidural block remains a debated question. After the introduction of the lumbar puncture by Quincke (1891) only 2 years after Bier's spinal anesthesia (1898), in 1900, Kreis pioneered the use of spinal anesthesia in six parturients for labor pain relief. The very frequent and severe complications related to spinal anesthesia motivated the physicians to investigate other approaches to the spinal cord and nerves, and the most logical was the epidural. Historically, the first approach to the epidural space was that of the caudal, preceding the lumbar, thoracic, and cervical ones. Nine years after the experience with the sacral approach described by Sicard and Chatelin in 1901, Stoeckel introduced the caudal epidural for labor pain relief and until the 1920s, caudal anesthesia was considered the safest route to the epidural space. Sicard and Forestier in 1921 described a technique to reach the lumbar epidural space for neuroradiological purposes and Pagés in the same year sensed that the needle should be stopped in the epidural space to produce a metameric anesthesia. In the early 1930s Dogliotti developed and disseminated the loss of resistance technique and Gutierrez discovered the hanging-drop technique. Graffagnino was the first to use the lumbar approach for labor analgesia while the continuous lumbar technique was introduced by Aburel in 1931, improving the practice of labor pain relief. He also started the

systematic investigation of the afferent innervation of the uterus completed by Cleland in 1933 and by Bonica in the 1950s. Finally, Bonica and Bromage (1954) took the practice of epidural anesthesia into the modern era. In their books the epidural block technique is described in an exhaustive way based on their great personal experience and they remain today the major reference for every obstetric anesthesiologist.

1.1 Was the Very First a Spinal or an Epidural Anesthesia?

The beginning of modern local anesthesia may be traced to the late nineteenth century with the availability of the three elements necessary for its administration: a syringe, a needle, and a local anesthetic drug. The year 1885 may be considered the founding year of neuraxial anesthesia with the publication by Corning of the historical article entitled "Spinal anesthesia and local medication of the cord (1885)" [1], followed, only 1 year later, by the first textbook on local anesthesia, *Local Anesthesia in General Medicine and Surgery* (New York, 1886) [2].

James Leonard Corning (1855–1923), a New York neurologist, was born in Connecticut but received his medical education in Germany, graduating from the University of Wurzburg in 1878. The introduction of the hollow needle and the glass syringe by Alexander Wood

© Springer Nature Switzerland AG 2020
G. Capogna, *Epidural Technique In Obstetric Anesthesia*,
https://doi.org/10.1007/978-3-030-45332-9_1

(1817–1884) in 1853 and the clinical demonstration of the local anesthetic properties of cocaine by Karl Koller (1858–1944) in 1884 were the preliminary steps leading to Corning's research that he conducted using hydrochlorate of cocaine on both the peripheral and central nervous systems. He observed that subcutaneous injection of cocaine was associated with both vasoconstriction and local anesthesia and thus hypothesized that injecting cocaine solution into the subcutaneous tissues between two contiguous spinal processes would result in its uptake by veins afferent to the cord. He wrote: "I hoped to produce artificially a temporary condition of things analogous in its physiological consequences to the effects observed in transverse myelitis or after total section of the cord" [1].

At that time the aim of any injection was to deposit the drug as near as possible to the site on which it was desired to act. For example for many years physicians continued to consider morphine effective only if injected close to the painful lesions. In tune with this theory of the time, Corning aimed to deposit the cocaine in close contact with the cord, but at the same time was also searching for a method to avoid the risk of injuring it by puncture.

His first experiment involved injecting 20 minims (1.3 mL) of a 2% cocaine solution into the space between two inferior dorsal vertebrae of a young dog. Within 5 min he noted first incoordination and later weakness and anesthesia of the animal's hind legs which resolved completely in approximately 4 h. The effect did not spread to the forelegs and he attributed this fact "to the lethargy of the circulation at this point."

After this animal experience, he carried out his well-known experiment on man.

He had previously observed that in the lower thoracic region, the vertebral transverse processes lie at the same depth as the laminae which form the posterior boundary of the vertebral canal. He therefore first inserted the needle lateral to the midline until the point of the needle touched the transverse process, and then adjusted a marker located on the shaft of the needle to the skin level. The needle was then reinserted, this time in the midline between the two spines, not quite up to the marker to prevent a too deep an insertion and therefore a possible cord injury (Fig. 1.1).

In a man who suffered "spinal weakness" and "seminal incontinence," he injected 30 minims (2 mL) of 3% cocaine into the T11/12 interspinous space. No effect was noted within 6–8 min and he repeated the injection. Ten minutes later

Fig. 1.1 The method Corning used to deposit the drug as near as possible to the desired site

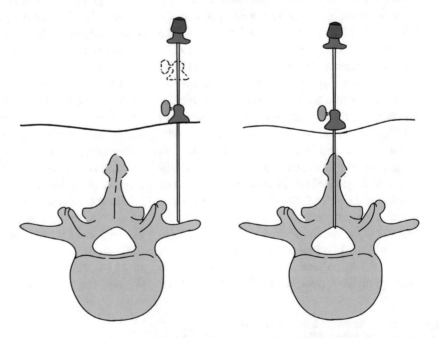

the subject remarked that his legs felt "sleepy" and Corning could demonstrate "greatly impaired" sensitivity to pinprick in the legs, genitalia, and lumbar region which lasted over 15–20 min. No motor weakness or gait disturbance was noted.

Corning did not mention the ligamentum flavum nor the dura mater. In addition he introduced the needle with a charged syringe already attached to the needle, and injected the solution without any previous aspiration, so preventing him from noticing the possible appearance of cerebrospinal fluid in the syringe.

The man made a full recovery but, interestingly, Corning recorded that he complained of headache and vertigo the next morning.

Whether in his first human experiment Corning had obtained, however unknowingly, true spinal anesthesia or merely had produced epidural anesthesia remains a debated question. It seems plausible that Corning's early experimentation resulted in effects more similar to an epidural anesthetic although with signs of some inadvertent dural puncture. Corning's dose of local anesthetic was eight times higher than the doses of the same drug successfully used by Gustav Bier 14 years later for his spinal anesthesia [3]. Yet, the onset of analgesia in Corning's patient was slower and the ultimate sensory level lower. In addition it is certain that Corning's experiment was based on faulty physiological and anatomical premises, since he believed that cocaine injected into the region between two spinous processes would be absorbed by the circulation and transferred to the substance of the cord.

Even in his later experiences, Corning appears to have regarded his intentional intrathecal injections only as a tool to alleviate the existing pain while overlooking its possibilities in surgery.

In his *Pain in its neuropathical relations* (Philadelphia, 1884) [4] under the heading "The irrigation of the cauda equina with medicinal fluids," he wrote: "I became impressed with the desirability of introducing remedies directly into spinal canal with a view to producing still more powerful impressions on the cord, and more especially on its lower segment." He introduced a needle through a small introducer between the L2 and L3 interspace deliberately to perform a

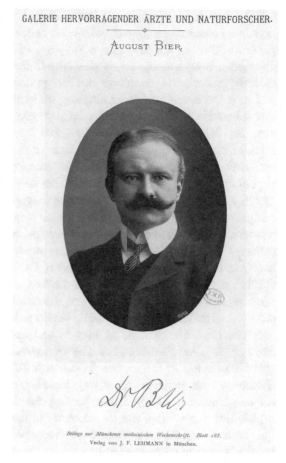

Fig. 1.2 August Karl Gustav Bier (1861–1949) (from Bibliotèque Interuniversitaire de Santé, Paris. Open Licence)

lumbar puncture to medicate the cord because of "spinal irritation," but this was 3 years after the technique of lumbar puncture had been described in detail by **Heinrich Irenaeus Quincke** (1842–1922) in 1891 [5].

Unfortunately the work of Corning on clinical local analgesia attracted little attention and had no influence on clinical practice, but his investigations on cocainization of the cord antedated Bier's classic and highly influential experiments by 18 years.

In fact it was 14 years after Corning's first publication that **August Karl Gustav Bier** (1861–1949) (Fig. 1.2), a German surgeon, published the first reports of successful spinal anesthesia in surgery: *"Versuche uber Cocainisirung des Ruckenmarks"* (Experiments with cocainization of the spinal cord)

[3]. On August 16, 1898, Bier injected 15 mg of intrathecal cocaine in a 34-year-old worker undergoing resection of a tuberculous ankle joint. His description is remarkable for its similarity to the modern process: he described positioning the patient in the lateral position, infiltrating the skin and subcutaneous tissues with the cocaine solution, and observing the flow of cerebrospinal fluid from a long hollow needle before injection of the anesthetic solution into the dural sac. He went on to perform five more spinal anesthetics in the same month. Complete anesthesia was achieved only in one patient; five patients could still sense touch or pressure, but not pain. Furthermore in four of these patients, Bier reported complications including back and leg pain, vomiting, and headache. Even at this early stage, he had associated the loss of cerebrospinal fluid with headache, and discussed the risks of toxicity. Within the same publication Bier describes the attempts of himself and his assistant, Dr. Otto Hildebrandt, to deliver cocaine spinal anesthetics to one another. Sensation in Dr. Hildebrandt was tested in various ways including a needle pushed down to the femur, burning cigars, avulsion of pubic hairs, and strong blows to the tibia with an iron hammer, none of which resulted in pain. In spite of promising results, complications were recorded including paresthesia in a lower limb and the loss of "much" cerebrospinal fluid. Bier reported that subsequently he experienced a severe headache, associated with dizziness which was relieved completely by lying flat for a total of 9 days [3].

Only 2 years after Bier's spinal anesthesia, in 1900, **Oskar Kreis** (1872–1958), a gynecologist and obstetrician from Basel, pioneered the use of spinal anesthesia in six parturients for labor pain relief. He used cocaine as a local anesthetic, and all but one patient had nausea, vomiting, and severe postpartum headache.

1.2   The First Epidural Approach: The Caudal

The very frequent and severe complications related to spinal anesthesia such as hypotension, nausea, vomiting, postdural puncture headache, and meningeal irritation motivated physicians in Europe and the Americas to investigate other approaches to the spinal cord and nerves, and the most logical being the epidural.

Historically, the first approach to the epidural space was the caudal, preceding the lumbar, thoracic, and cervical approaches.

In 1901, two French physicians, working independently of one another in Paris, **Jean-Athanase Sicard** (1872–1929), neurologist and radiologist, and **Fernard Cathelin** (1873–1945) claimed the birthright of discovering epidural analgesia.

Sicard had released the first publication on epidural injections. In an article entitled "*Les injections mèdicamenteuses extra durales par voie sacro-coccygienne*" (sacro-coccygeal extradural drug injection) [6], on 20 April 1901, he discussed spinal anesthesia with cocaine and commented on the severe headaches, nausea, and vomiting that were produced postoperatively. He then went on to describe his caudal epidural technique in the dog, a human cadaver, and nine patients with pain who had all obtained immediate analgesia. He stated that this technique should replace spinal anesthesia.

One week later, Cathelin presented his work to the Society of Biology in Paris and stressed that he had been working and experimenting with this new method since 5 February 1901. Evidence was given by his chief, Professor Lejars, as to the truth of this statement. His address was entitled "*Une novelle voie d'injection rachidienne. Methode des injections epidurales par le procede du canal sacre. Applications a l'homme*" (A new spinal injection route. Method of epidural injection by the sacral canal method. Applications to man) [7]. He described the caudal injection of cocaine 1% into dogs, and he demonstrated with Indian ink that his injections were limited to the extradural space. In February 1901 he performed caudal block on four patients who were undergoing surgery for hernia repair, but with imperfect results. He stated that further study was needed but he thought that the technique would be useful for surgical operations, to produce analgesia for painful deliveries, inoperable rectal carcinoma, and hemorrhoidal fissures. Controversy ensued, but in the final analysis Sicard relinquished the discovery to the young Cathelin. It subsequently became apparent that Cathelin was worthy of this generous gesture, since he produced 22 publications and notes about this new method. In 1902 he published his thesis on epidural injections and submitted it for the Doctorate in Medicine. This work was obviously the basis for further research. He refuted Corning's priority in using the epidural space and 20 years after the discovery which he had claimed, he described spinal anesthesia as the "poor relation of my method." It must be remembered that cocaine was the only local anesthetic available initially and was sometimes too toxic in the concentrations required to produce analgesia similar to spinal anesthesia.

In the year 1905 the German chemist **Alfred Einhorn** (1856–1917) synthesized procaine, and gave it the trade name of Novocaine, from the Latin nov- (new) and -caine, the common ending for alkaloids used as anesthetic. The new drug was promptly used for caudal anesthesia since it was less toxic, more effective, and more stable than the previously used cocaine.

Walter Stoeckel (1871–1961), professor of gynecology in Marburg, with a special interest in gynecological urology, injected cocaine solutions into the epidural space, through the sacral hiatus. Stoeckel described a series of 141 cases of obstetric caudal epidural analgesia in an article entitled *Uber Sakrale Anasthesie* in 1909 [8]. According to the English translation of this original paper, edited by one of the pioneers of epidural anesthesia, Andrew Doughty [9], he wrote: "In 18 cases there was no noticeable beneficial effect and in a further 12 the relief of pain was minimal. Positive relief was obtained in the remaining 111 cases but to varying degrees. It became apparent that labour pain is not a single entity but is made up of two distinct components which became recognizable by our experience with sacral anaesthesia [...] After an effective sacral block the pain of uterine contraction disappears or at least diminishes and becomes quite tolerable [...] We have obtained complete relief or reduction to a tolerable degree of the back pain in 72 cases and of both back and hypogastric pain in 39 cases. The considerable degree of relief was evidenced by

the behavior of the mothers in whom the pains were no longer accompanied by loud crying and rolling about in bed; the contractions could then only be perceived by abdominal palpation [...] Pain sensitivity in the perineum was mostly, but not always, obtunded when tested with a needle. Thus the passage of the head through the vulva was painless in nine cases and only very slightly painful in 16. Three women were delivered by forceps and two had perineal tears sutured quite painlessly. In two other cases, sacral anaesthesia was insufficient for the application of forceps and these patients had to be helped with a few drops of chloroform. In many cases there was a marked relaxation of the pelvic floor musculature. [...] In 23 cases the contractions became weaker and less frequent and this depressive effect was especially noticeable if the injection had been given too early in labour; in one case the contractions ceased with the pain and did not return for 4 days. [...] However, if labour had been well established, neither the uterine contractions nor the expulsive forces were affected as a general rule."

In the early 1900s through to the 1920s, caudal anesthesia was considered the safest route to the epidural space. Operations utilizing epidural anesthesia were usually limited to the region of the body supplied by the cauda equina. Attempts to push the block higher by using larger volumes of anesthetic or changing the patient's position were not always successful.

However, **Robert Emmett Farr** (1875–1932), surgeon in Minneapolis, was able to produce anesthesia to the level of the nipples injecting volumes up to 120 mL of local anesthetic introduced through the caudal space. In his paper, *"Sacral Anesthesia,"* published in 1926 [10], Farr described his cadaveric experiments. Using contrast dye and X-rays, he showed dissemination of contrast from the epidural space via the epidural foramina. He also described the spread of contrast to the level of the cervical vertebrae when volumes greater than 80 ml were introduced through the caudal canal.

Caudal sacral analgesia became popular in obstetric analgesia in the first 20–40 years of the twentieth century. However it had at the very least a discrete failure rate even in the best hands, due to both the variations in the anatomy of the caudal canal and the difficulty, often the impossibility, of identifying the caudal hiatus in the parturient at term. In addition while caudal analgesia was able to produce successful perineal and second-stage analgesia, it could not provide pain relief from uterine contraction unless large doses were used, with the risk of toxicity and a slowing down of the labor process.

1.3   Lumbar Epidural

As early as 1921, two French radiologists, **Jean Sicard** (1872–1929) **and Jacques Forestier** (1890–1978), described a "loss of resistance" to syringe injection as a spinal needle was advanced through the lumbar ligaments. They were injecting radiographic contrast (lipiodol) to treat chronic lumbar and sciatic pain while studying spinal canal abnormalities and described this "loss of resistance" as the entry of the needle tip into the epidural space. In the course of this procedure they accidentally injected a few millimeters of lipiodol in the subarachnoid space, producing a myelography with no arachnoideal adverse reaction [11]. However, both were of the opinion that lumbar and thoracic epidural space was not suitable for the diffusion of the injected solutions, due to the presumed presence of tough septa and for the easy diffusion of the liquid itself through the vertebral foramina. In the same year, **Fidel Pagés Miravé** (1886–1923) (Fig. 1.3), a Spanish military surgeon, was the first person to perform epidural anesthesia by the lumbar route.

In his paper *Anestesia Metamérica* (Metameric Anesthesia) which was published in March 1921 simultaneously in the *Revista Espaniola de Cirugia* [12] and in *the Revista de Sanidad Militar* [13], he described his original idea: *"En el mes de noviembre del pasado año, al practicar una raquianestesia, tuve la idea de detener la cánula en pleno conducto raquídeo, antes de atravesar la duramadre, y me propuse bloquear las raíces fuera del espacio meníngeo, y antes de atravesar los agujeros de conjunción, puesto que la punta de la aguja había atravesado el ligamento amarillo correspondiente."*

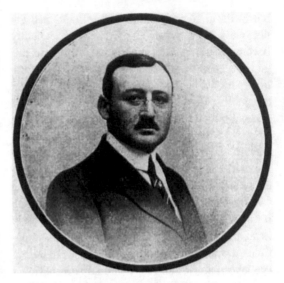

Fig. 1.3   Fidel Pagés Miravé (1886–1923) (from Lange JJ et al. (2007) Anaesthesia 49: 429–431, with permission)

This is the English translation of his original description of epidural anesthesia which relied on his feeling for the "snap" as the needle passed through the ligamentum flavum and entered the epidural space: "In November of last year, while I was carrying out spinal anesthesia, I had the idea of detaining the cannula with the spinal canal, before it penetrated the dura mater, and then blocking the roots outside the meningeal space before the needle traversed the corresponding foramina, since the point of the needle had traversed the corresponding yellow ligament. I abandoned the Stovaine that I had prepared, and in a sterilized capsule dissolved three tablets of Suprarenin Novocaine of series A (375 mg of Novocaine) in 25 mL of physiologic serum, and proceeded to inject it immediately through the cannula which was placed between the second and third lumbar vertebrae. Hypoesthesia became accentuated progressively, and within 20 min after injection we decided that it was permissible to start the operation. We carried out radical repair of a right inguinal hernia without the least discomfort to the patient."

After this, he described his experience with this technique in 43 patients (including upper abdominal operations) (Fig. 1.4).

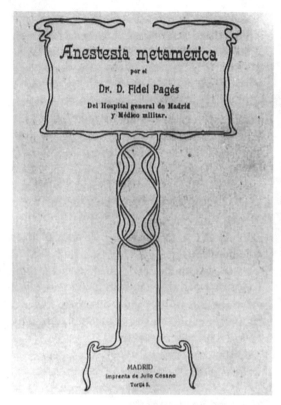

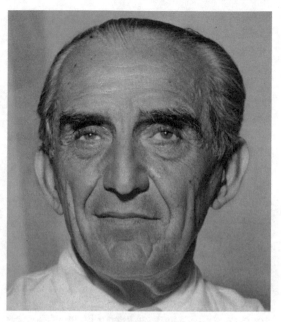

Fig. 1.5 Achille Mario Dogliotti (1897–1966)

Fig. 1.4 First page of the paper "Anestesia Metamerica" published by Fidel Pagés in 1921 (from Lange JJ et al. (2007) Anaesthesia 49: 429–431, with permission)

Unfortunately his work did not circulate in the scientific world at that time, since he published only in Spanish and he did not present his work at any congress. In addition his premature and unexpected death certainly contributed to the lack of dissemination of his work.

Independently of Pagés, an Italian surgeon, Achille Mario Dogliotti who did not previously know about Pagés' work described epidural anesthesia through the lumbar route in 1931. A controversy as to who was the first to discover lumbar epidural anesthesia consequently arose. Dogliotti, as president of the International College of Surgeons, attended numerous conferences and published in the English language, facilitating the diffusion of his technique. Dogliotti learnt later of the work of Pagés and acknowledged him as the first to develop and describe the lumbar epidural approach [14].

However, whereas Pagés used a tactile approach to identify the epidural space, Dogliotti was the first to identify it by using the loss of resistance technique.

Achille Mario Dogliotti (1897–1966) (Fig. 1.5), professor of surgery in Modena, Catania, and Turin, was an innovator of Italian surgery, having developed one of the first heart-lung machines. He was also a pioneer in the X-ray techniques of the biliary tract and responsible for the organization of the first blood bank in Italy. He may be considered the "father" of modern epidural anesthesia since he first described the modern loss of resistance technique that overcame the main obstacle to the advancement of lumbar and thoracic epidural anesthesia due to the inability to reproducibly identify the epidural space at those levels.

We can consider the "birth certificate" of lumbar epidural anesthesia the lecture Dogliotti gave on April 18, 1931, at the meeting of the Società Piemontese di Chirurgia (Piemontese Society of Surgery) which was entitled *"Un promettente metodo di anestesia tronculare in studio: la rachianestesia peridurale segmentaria"* (A study on a promising method of troncular anesthesia: segmental peridural rachianesthesia) [15].

As he explained during his lecture at the XIth Annual Congress of Anesthesiologists, in

New York City in October 1932 [16], Dogliotti was looking for an alternative to spinal anesthesia, since "inconveniences always complained about in spinal anesthesia, besides the decrease of blood pressure, are nausea and vomiting during the operation (about 30% of the cases), and postoperative headaches (about 10–20%)" and defined his epidural approach as "a regional anesthesia covering a large region which permits the obtaining for the upper and lower abdomen, for the extremities and for the thorax what the Cathelin epidural sacral anesthesia obtains for the perineum and pelvis."

After having recognized the relative difficulty of the lumbar epidural technique encountered in the past, Dogliotti explained how he had made it simple and reliable: "The technique has been made easy and simple by introducing the needle, connected with a syringe filled with physiological solution, slowly and exercising at the same time as the needle penetrates the yellow ligaments a constant and considerable pressure on the piston. While the needle is penetrating the yellow ligaments, a strong resistance to the injection of the liquid is felt. As soon as the needle pierces the ligaments and arrives in the peridural space, all resistance is at once removed and the liquid enters with every facility separating the dura mater from the peridural adipose tissue. The needle is thus in place and after having ascertained that there is no flow of either blood or cerebro-spinal fluid, the next procedure is the injection of the anesthetic which will diffuse itself in the peridural space" (Fig. 1.6).

Dogliotti's method of identification of the epidural space was a very important innovation that launched this valuable technique in the modern practice of anesthesiology. The previously described methods, such as that described by Pagés, were primarily tactile methods of identifying the epidural space, noting the "feel" of the needle tip as it passed through the ligamentum flavum, and this limited these techniques to the manually clever. Instead Dogliotti's technique was reproducible and easily learned. Dogliotti's Anesthesia Textbook was published in 1935 [17], was translated into English in 1939 [18], and contained an extensive and detailed chapter on epidural analgesia which also included all his exhaustive studies performed on this matter. Textbooks by American authors several years later contained only a short description of the technique, treating it as a novelty practiced only by those with special expertise.

Initial acceptance of epidural analgesia was therefore slow to develop in North America, although it gained early and wide acceptance in Europe and South America.

In the 1930s, **Alberto Guiterrez** (1892–1945) (Fig. 1.7), professor of surgery in Buenos Aires, used the epidural anesthesia technique from Pagés and Dogliotti and applied it for thousands of different operations. Concerned about general anesthesia accidents, Gutierrez turned to other alternatives. He first used spinal anesthesia, and then epidural anesthesia in an approach called at that time the "direct method" (loss of resistance). Occasionally, he used what was indicated as the

Fig. 1.6 Original Dogliotti's description of his loss of resistance technique: the syringe is held in one hand, the thumb of which applies a continued and uniform pressure to the piston (from [16] with permission)

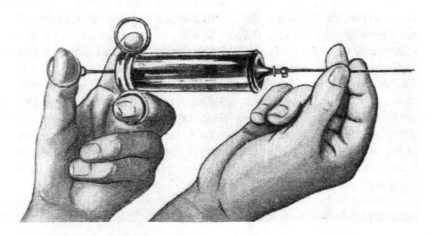

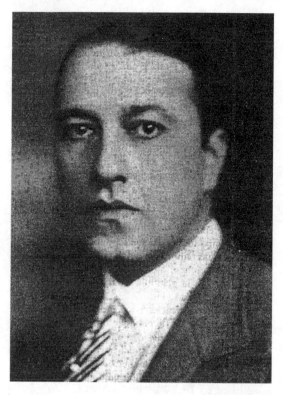

Fig. 1.7 Alberto Gutierrez (1892–1945) (from [19] with permission)

"indirect method," in which the needle was intentionally introduced into the dural sac, and then gradually withdrawn a few millimeters until the cerebrospinal fluid stopped dripping, assuming that at that moment, the bevel was as in the epidural space. Antonio Aldrete [19] describes the history of the Gutierrez discovery as follows: "One day in February 1933, Alberto Gutierrez was searching for the epidural space by use of the loss- of-resistance method with fluid. Apparently, while introducing the tip of the needle through the interspinous ligament and approaching the ligamentum flavum, he felt undue resistance, so he disconnected the syringe and noted that a drop of the fluid was left hanging from the hub. He did not reattach the syringe but continued to advance the needle, without touching the drop. As he continued to insert the needle very slowly, he suddenly noticed that the drop disappeared. He then reconnected the syringe and aspirated without obtaining fluid." After fractionated doses of 1% procaine without feeling resistance up to

15 mm, he was able to perform a painless saphenectomy. This observation was reported in an informal way in the periodical *el Dia Medico* on March 27, 1933 [20], and followed by a formal paper in the *Revista de Cirugia* [21]. Gutierrez reported that sometimes the drop did not hang, but rather a meniscus of fluid could be observed within the hub, in which case the needle must be advanced very slowly and injected only when the fluid could no longer be seen.

In 1938 Gutierrez published in his book *Extradural Anesthesia* [22] the updated experience of everyone he knew that was practicing epidural anesthesia, including Dogliotti who, at the time, had performed over 4000 cases.

Of interest were his attempts to find out about the negative pressure in the epidural space.

Gutierrez's way of using the negative epidural pressure as a marker of finding the epidural space by placing a drop of saline on the hub of the advancing needle became known as the sign of the hanging drop.

In 1936 **Charles Odom** (1909–1988), director of surgical services at the Charity Hospital of New Orleans, substituted a capillary tube for the hanging drop as follows [23]: "I cut a small glass adapter commonly used to connect a rubber infusion hose to an infusion needle, in half and connected it to the spinal needle after it had been engaged in the interspinous ligament. The ground glass tip of the adapter made the connection air-tight. The lumen of the adapter was then filled with sterile solution. This small glass cylinder with the enclosed fluid made a very delicate indicator. The smaller the bore of the cylinder the more delicate it becomes. This indicator is very easily sterilized and is far less cumbersome to use than the spinal manometers or U tubes used in some of the European clinics." Odom performed a large number of surgeries with this technique including two cesarean sections in women with tuberculosis.

Odom suggested that the epidural space is a potential space in the erect posture and that it only comes into existence when the spine is flexed and the two layers of the dura mater separate. As the anterior wall of the vertebral column does not flex as much as the posterior wall, a space is created between them and as this space is formed from no space at all, a vacuum will be created. This vacuum will slowly dissipate owing to an influx of venous blood until atmospheric pressure is achieved.

In the same hospital **Peter Graffagnino**, a gynecologist, "attempted to add to the anesthetic armamentarium of the obstetrician another procedure, epidural anesthesia, which we have thus far administered to 76 patients" with this publication of February 1939 [24], in which he became the first to report the use of lumbar epidural block for labor analgesia, performed according to Odom's technique. In his conclusions he stated: "The anesthetic can be administered to all patients in the childbearing age. All major operative obstetrical procedures can be performed under this form of anesthesia safely and with the conscious cooperation of the patient."

The era of epidural indicators had started, and a number of visual and mechanical devices were developed to help the physician to identify the epidural space.

Massey Dawkins (1905–1975), consultant anesthetist at the University College, London, pioneer of epidurals, the first to administer it in the UK in 1942, in 1963 wrote an extensive review of the main devices in use at that time [25] (Figs. 1.8 and 1.9): "(1) In the Iklè syringe the pressure of the thumb is replaced by a spring which drives the piston forward as soon as the epidural space is entered. (2) In 1935 Macintosh modified this spring loading on the piston by applying spring pressure to a blunt trocar inside the epidural needle. This trocar will not normally pierce the dura. While the needle is traversing the interspinous ligaments, the distal end of the trocar projects from the hub of the needle. When the point of the needle enters the space, a hidden spring in the hub of the needle drives the trocar forward and the distal end of the trocar disappears into the hub. This is an excellent device as the weight of the needle is unaltered and there are two wings protruding on either side of the hub which make for ease in handling … No data concerning the efficiency of this device have been recorded in the literature. (3) A simpler device, also introduced by Macintosh, consists of a balloon distended by air which is plugged into the hub of the needle … Directly the advancing needle enters the space, the balloon will deflate. It is advisable to use a fresh balloon for each case in order to avoid leaks. Although the balloon is widely used, no details of its efficiency have been published, but enquiries among colleagues who use it have established that in 506 cases there was a dural puncture rate of 6.7%. (4) In 1956 Zelenka suggested that the tactile and visual techniques could be combined in one device. He took a U shaped manometer containing bubbles of air in sterile water and fitted a tap at the distal end into which a distended balloon could be plugged. When the needle was in the interspinous ligament the device was attached and the tap opened. Now as soon as the space was entered the meniscus received an impulse of positive pressure from behind which helped to overcome the 19% failure rate of the visual technique alone. There are however no recorded details of the efficiency of this device. (5) In 1958 the above device was simplified by Brooks who took an Odom's indicator, heated the distal end, sealed it and then blew a small bulb in it. If a bubble of air in saline is placed in the capillary tube and the indicator is plugged into the hub of the epidural needle and the bulb is then heated, the air within it expands and provides a positive pressure behind the meniscus. This exceedingly simple device works well in practice and in my own experience converts a success rate with Odom's indicator alone of 73% to one of 90%."

1.4   Continuous Lumbar Epidural

Clinicians realized that to provide continuous anesthesia for long-lasting surgical procedures, there had to be a way to repeatedly inject local anesthetics.

As with the epidural single-shot technique, the continuous method also used this technique first starting from the caudal and spinal route, the lumbar approach only being considered a few years later on.

Eugen Bogdan Aburel (1899–1975) (Fig. 1.10), Romanian professor in obstetrics and

Fig. 1.8 Various types of epidural indicators (1935–1958) (from [25] with permission)

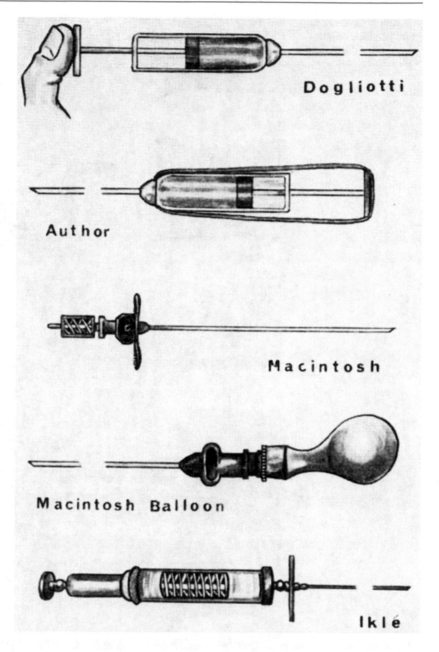

gynecology, and a pioneer in obstetric analgesia, in 1931 presented his technique of *"anesthèsie locale continue (prolonguèe) en obstètrique"* (continuous local anesthesia in obstetrics) [26]. His technique for insertion of the catheter through the needle withdrawing the needle over it and positioning the catheter is very similar to what is in use today. Curelaru [27] describes Aburel's description of his technique as follows: "Firstly, introduce the needle at the selected level (epidural, lumbo-aortic): inject 30 mL of cinchocaine (Percaine) 0.5%; introduce through the needle a soft catheter (similar to ureteric catheters); remove the needle with the catheter left in situ: finally, apply a dressing above the catheter. If repeated injections are required, they could be performed with a fine needle through the catheter left in situ ... Through ... the needle-catheter approach, it becomes possible to obtain prolonged local anaesthesia in obstetrics.

Fig. 1.9 Various types of epidural indicators (1935–1958) (from [25] with permission)

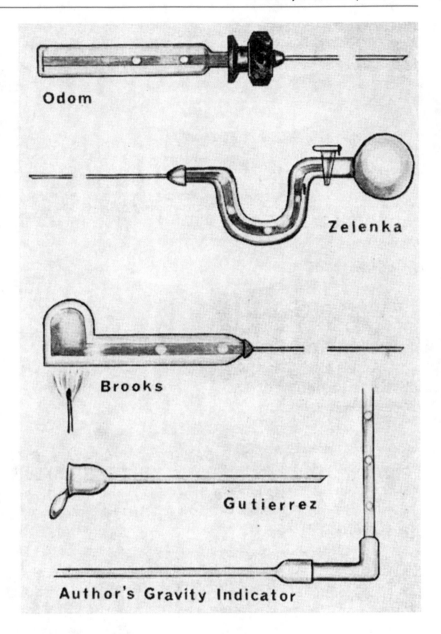

This approach should no longer be considered experimental but as an everyday procedure." The catheter used by Aburel was made of flexible silk and resembled a ureteric catheter. Aburel also began a systematic investigation of the afferent innervation of the uterus by meticulous anatomical dissection and sharp clinical observation in parallel with the analogue researches (1927–1933) of Cleland on this subject in the USA. However, since his publications were written in French [28, 29], they went unnoticed by overseas colleagues.

John Cleland (1898–1980), from the University of Oregon, used paravertebral block and low caudal analgesia to "present experimental proof via visceromotor reflexes of the location of these paths in the dog, to correlate these findings in man, to explain the error of conclusions hitherto accepted, and to demonstrate that the pain of uterine contraction may be abolished without affecting the contractions by paravertebral block of only two adjacent nerves" [30]. Cleland concluded in his paper of 1933 [30] that the sensory afferents from the uterus and cervix that transmit

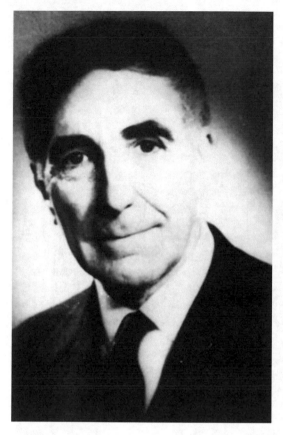

Fig. 1.10 Eugen Bogdan Aburel (1899–1975) (from [26] with permission)

pain during the first stage of labor enter the spinal cord T11 and T12 and that the second stage of labor is primarily somatic in nature and it is transmitted through the sacral nerves.

William Lemmon (1896–1974) published preliminarily in 1940 [31] and more extensively in 1944 [32] the description of a 17G or 18G nickel-silver alloy malleable needle (Fig. 1.11). The needle was placed in the subarachnoid space, was bent at the skin surface, and was attached to rubber tubing through which local anesthetic solution was injected when required. The patient lay on a mattress and table that had a hole placed so as to accommodate the protruding needle (Fig. 1.12).

Robert Hingson (1913–1996), Chief of Anesthesia of the Marine Hospital at Staten Island, USA, after trying malleable needles inserted caudally, used continuous epidural anesthesia by the caudal route, injecting local anesthetics through ureteral catheters. With his Chief Obstetrician colleague, **Waldo Edwards**

(1905–1981), they decided to combine the advantages of continuous spinal analgesia with the safety, simplicity, and effectiveness of sacral epidural block. Securing the hub of the malleable needle to rigid rubber tubing, the analgesic agent could be introduced with the patient in her hospital room, uninterrupted during transfer to the delivery site, and easily maneuvered for preparation, delivery, and, if necessary, episiotomy. Of course the needle was left in the caudal canal and the patient labored in the decubitus position. In their paper published in JAMA in 1942 [33] they wrote: "since that time we have managed the entire course of six hundred labors and deliveries with this method without restoring to any other form of anesthesia. We believe that continuous caudal analgesia has opened a new medical horizon to the profession comparable to that developed … with continuous spinal anesthesia … We would emphasize that with our method the drug producing the analgesia is continuously bathing the nerve trunks of the sacral and lumbar plexuses within the peridural space. Consequently the patient is still able to move the lower extremities throughout labor, and uterine contractions continue without impediment."

Edward B. Tuohy (1908–1959), in the 1940s, was aware of the early clinical work by Pagés and Dogliotti on epidural blocks, but he was particularly interested in continuous spinal anesthesia [34]. He replaced the sharp previously used needle with a needle that had been designed by **Ralph L. Huber** (1890–1953), a Seattle dentist. Huber's needle had a directional tip, which allowed the direction of the catheter as it exited the needle tip.

Although Huber intended this needle for intravenous and tissue injections, Tuohy recognized that the directional point might facilitate the placement of spinal catheters. In addition, he added a stylet hoping to further decrease the risk of skin plugging.

But it was **Pio Manuel Martinez Curbelo** (1905–1962), not Tuohy, who realized how the directional needle might facilitate the placement of epidural catheters and who may be considered the initiator of continuous lumbar epidural anesthesia. Curbelo visited Tuohy at the Mayo Clinic in November 1946. He observed Tuohy using his

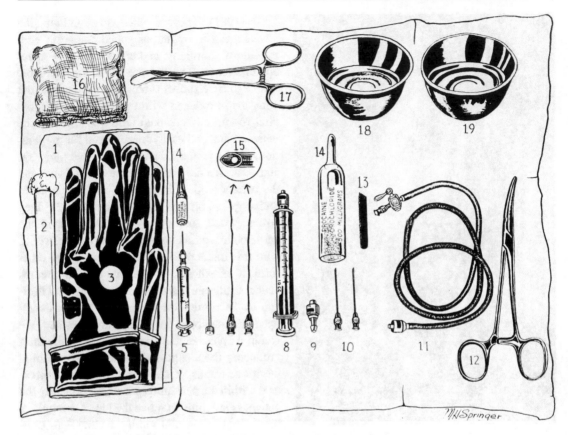

Fig. 1.11 Tray for continuous spinal anesthesia (1944) (from [32] with permission)

recently developed needle to allow for the insertion of ureteral catheters intrathecally and noted that by injecting small, fractionated doses of local anesthetics repeatedly, long-term analgesia could be achieved. On January 1947, at the Hospital Municipal de la Havana, he inserted a catheter into the lumbar epidural space in a 40-year-old woman about to have a laparotomy for removal of a giant ovarian cyst. He found the epidural space by the "loss of resistance" method, then passed a ureteral catheter through the needle, and then injected 1% procaine, followed by a supplemental dose 40 min later. He announced his success in a meeting of the Surgical Society of La Habana [35]. Alderete [36] reports his description made at the joint IARS and ICA International Congress in New York in September 1947: "The guide is introduced up to one cm from the tip of the catheter, which is inserted into the needle 9.5 cm, then placing the index finger of the left hand at the entry point of the needle into the skin and holding its hub with the left thumb and middle fingers,

the catheter is advanced with the right hand one more cm and the guide was removed one cm at a time, alternating this move with the advancing of the catheter, the same distance, until 12.5 cm indicating that the catheter is 3 cm in the epidural space. Slowly, the guide is removed and the 23 gauge needle, connected to a syringe is adapted to the catheter … A wide strip of sterile adhesive tape is applied over the entire length of catheter fixing it to the skin of the back making it accessible for ulterior supplementary doses; thereafter, the patient is placed in the supine position."

Curbelo used the "Pages-Dogliotti method of the loss of resistance" to identify the epidural space utilizing the 2 cc syringe containing 1.5 cc of normal saline. Occasionally he lubricated the outside wall of the needle with sterile Vaseline and advanced it millimeter by millimeter. In addition, he was known to place a drop of chloroform on the plunger of the syringe to obtain optimal seal while allowing free movement. Interestingly he recommended to always "feel the three open-

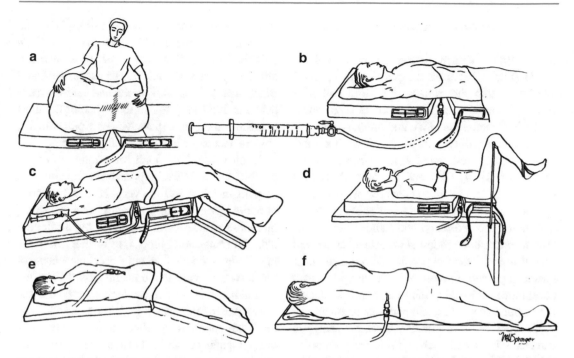

Fig. 1.12 Special mattress for continuous spinal anesthesia (1944) (from [32] with permission). (**a**) position of patient on special mattress for spinal puncture. (**b**) patient lying on back, with opening in mattress for adjusting needle. (**c**) patient in position for operation, showing syringe in sterile towel. Syringe and towel are fastened to mattress by towel clip. Strap on side of mattress is buckled during operation. (**d**) patient in perineal position. Lower half of mattress is detached. (**e**) patient in prone position for operations on back, anal region or posterior surface of extremities. (**f**) patient in Sim's position. Needle is bent at skin and fastened with adhesive. No special mattress is needed for the last two positions

ing steps, when the needle approached it, when it contacted it and finally when it penetrated" the ligamentum flavum, perceiving then a sudden disappearance of the resistance.

Charles Flowers (1920–1999) of the J Hopkins University in Baltimore was convinced that the work of Dogliotti evidenced that the lumbar peridural space could be used for the relief of obstetric pain. He published in August 1949 "Continuous peridural anesthesia and analgesia for labor, delivery and cesarean section" [37]. In this paper Flowers described his lumbar epidural loss of resistance technique using air, as follows: "When the dense ligamentum flavum has been entered, one pauses and tests the ease with which two cubic centimeters of air can be introduced into the ligament with a small syringe. When an attempt is made to inject air into the ligamentum flavum, the plunger of the syringe rebounds quickly. However, when air is injected into the peridural space, the plunger of the syringe literally falls into place. As the needle is advanced through the ligamentum flavum, frequent minute air tests are made with a small syringe to determine when the area of negative pressure in the peridural space is entered. Often this entrance is evident by the release of resistance that is felt when the blunt 16-gage Tuohy needle passes through the dense ligamentum flavum and enters the peridural space. When the Tuohy needle has been properly placed and there is no aspiration of spinal fluid, a plastic tube is introduced through the needle into the peridural space. The tubing is passed cephalad to the twelfth thoracic interspace for patients in early labor or about to undergo cesarean section. It is introduced caudal ward to the fourth lumbar space for patients in well-established labor."

In this paper Flowers reported 37 cases of cesarean section and 72 cases of labor analgesia conducted under continuous lumbar anesthesia and interestingly he noted that "whether peridural anesthesia is used for labor or cesarean section, one must always realize that the exact dose and time interval depends upon the somatic level of each patient."

1.5   Modern Epidural Analgesia

In the 1950s, **Philip Raikes Bromage** (1920–2013) (Fig. 1.13) took the practice of epidural anesthesia into the modern era. Born and educated in London, he became professor in anesthesia in Canada, the USA, and Saudi Arabia.

He published two major single-author textbooks on epidural anesthesia: *Spinal Epidural Analgesia* (1954) [38] and *Epidural Analgesia* (1978) [39]. The latter text covered all aspects of epidural anesthesia at the time of publication and it remains the reference book and a very valuable resource even today. It promoted safety and scientific basis for the practice of regional anesthesia. It played a pivotal role in the widespread acceptance and utilization of epidural analgesia for surgery, obstetrics, and pain management.

But the birth of modern obstetric analgesia can easily be traced back to **John Joseph Bonica** (1917–1994) (Fig. 1.14), an Italian-American physician, the father of the field of pain control, who devoted his career to the study of pain, establishing it as a multidisciplinary field. He created residency programs, chaired departments, wrote standard texts in the field, and had his work published in numerous languages. Among his huge number of publications, his masterpiece is *The Management of Pain* published for the first time in 1953 [40] and followed by numerous editions. His paper *"Peridural Block: analysis of 3637 cases and review,"* published in 1957 [41], is still today one of the most beautiful, in-depth, exhaustive descriptions of the epidural technique in all its practical aspects.

Bonica traced the path for a rational, reproducible, and effective approach for the abolition of pain in labor and delivery. He used a series of nerve blocks of various nociceptive pathways, including paracervical, segmental epidural, caudal, and trans-sacral blocks, to further refine the knowledge—due to Cleland's previous work—of the nerve pathways that transmit labor pain to the central nervous system. He demonstrated that the upper part of the cervix and lower uterine segment are supplied by afferents that accompany the sympathetic nerve through the uterine and cervical plexus; the inferior, middle, and superior hypogastric plexuses; and the aortic plexuses.

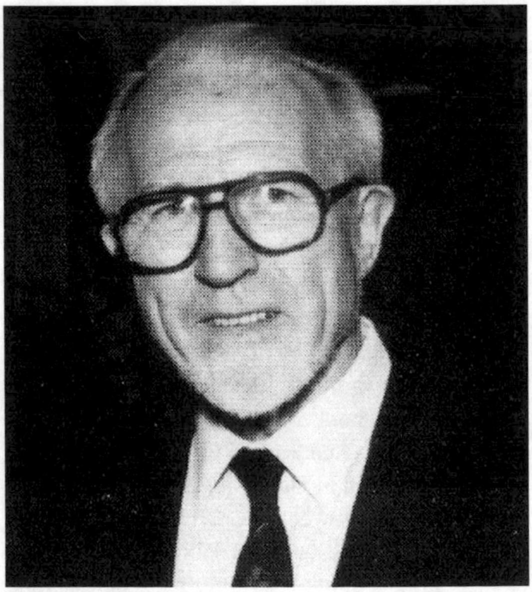

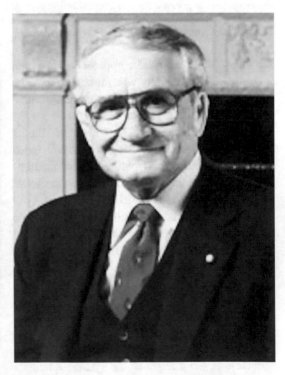

Fig. 1.13 Philip Raikes Bromage (1920–2013) (from Douglas (2013) IJOA 22:272, with permission)

Fig. 1.14 John Joseph Bonica (1917–1994)

In his *Principles and Practice of Obstetric Analgesia and Anesthesia* (1967 and 1995) [42, 43] the epidural block technique, as it may be used for labor analgesia, is described in a thorough and exhaustive way in accordance with his great personal experience and remains today the major reference for every obstetric anesthesiologist.

References

1. Corning JL. Spinal anaesthesia and local medication of the cord. N Y Med J. 1885;42:483–5.
2. Corning JL. Local anesthesia. New York: Appleton; 1886.
3. Bier A. Versuche uber Cocainisirung des Ruckenmarks. Deutsche Zeitschrift fur Chirurgie. 1899;51:361, translated in the "classical file" survey of Anesthesiology 1962; 6: 352.
4. Corning JL. Pain in its neuro-pathological diagnostic, medico legal, and neuro therapeutic relations. Philadelphia: JB Lippincott; 1894.
5. Quinke HI. Die Lumbarpunction des Hydrocephalus. Berl Klin Wochenschr. 1891;28:929–31.
6. Sicard A. Les injections mèdicamenteuses extra durales par voie sacro-coccygienne. C R Soc Biol Paris. 1901;53:396.
7. Cathelin F. Une nouvelle voie d'injection rachidienne; Méthodes des injections épidurales par le procédé du canal sacré. Applications àl'homme. C R Soc Biol. 1901;53:452–3.
8. Stoekel W. Uber sakrale Anasthesie. Zentralblatt fur Gynekologie. 1909;33:1–15.
9. Doughty A. Walter Stoeckel (1871-1961). A pioneer of regional analgesia in obstetrics. Anaesthesia. 1990;45:468–71.
10. Farr RE. Sacral anesthesia. Arch Surg. 1926;12:715–26.
11. Sicard JA, Forestier J. Mèthode radiographiqueration de la cavitè èpidurale par le lipiodol. Rev Neurol. 1921;137:1264–6.
12. Pagès F. Anesthesia metamerica. Rev Esp Chir. 1921;3:3–30.
13. Pagès F. Anestesia metamerica. Rev Sanid Mil. 1921;11:351–96.
14. Dogliotti AM. Trattato di Anestesia. Torino: UTET; 1946. p. 459.
15. Dogliotti AM. Un promettente metodo di anestesia tronculare in studio: la rachianestesia peridurale segmentaria. Bollettino della Società Piemontese di Chirurgia. 1931;I:385–99.
16. Dogliotti AM. Research and clinical observations on spinal anesthesia with special reference to the peridural technique. Anesth Analg. 1933;12:59–65.
17. Dogliotti AM. Trattato di Anestesia- Narcosi- Anestesia Locali, Regionali, Spinali. Torino: UTET; 1935.
18. Dogliotti AM. Anesthesia narcosis, local, regional, spinal. Chicago: SB Debour; 1939.
19. Aldrete JA, Auad OA, Gutierrez VP, et al. Alberto Gutierrez and the hanging drop. RAPM. 2005;30:397–404.
20. Gutierrez A. El valor de la aspiracion liquida en el espacio epidural en la anestesia peridural. Dia Medico. 1933.
21. Gutierrez A. Valor de la aspiracion liquida en el espacio peridural, en la anestesia peridural. Rev Cirugia. 1933;12:225–7.
22. Gutierrez A. Anestesia extradural. Buenos Aires: Imprenta; 1938.
23. Odom C. Epidural anesthesia. Am J Surg. 1936;34:547–58.
24. Graffagnino P, Syler KW. Epidural anesthesia in obstetrics. Anesth Analg. 1939;18:48–51.
25. Dowkins M. The identification of the epidural space. Anaesthesia. 1963;18:66–77.
26. Aburel E. L'anesthèsie locale (prolongèe) en obstètrique. Bullettin de la Sociètè d'Obstètrique et Gynècologie de Paris. 1931;20:35–27.
27. Curelaru I, Sandu L. Eugen Bogdan Aburel. The pioneer of regional anesthesia for pain relief in childbirth. Anaesthesia. 1982;37:663–9.
28. Aburel E. La topographie et le mecanisrne des doulerus de l'acouchement avant la periode d'expulsion. Comptes Rendus de la Sociète de Biologie de Paris. 1930;15:902–4.
29. Aburel E. Contribution à l'etude des voies nerveuses sensitives de l'uterus. Comptes Rendus de la Sociète de Biologie de Paris. 1930;25:297–9.
30. Cleland JPG. Paravertebral anaesthesia in obstetrics. Experimental and clinical basis. In: Survey of anesthesiology (1981). 1933;25:341–353.
31. Lemmon WT. A method for continuous spinal anesthesia. Ann Surg. 1940;111:141–4.
32. Lemmon WT. Continuous spinal anesthesia. Observations on 2000 cases. Ann Surg. 1944;120:129–42.
33. Hingson RA, Edwards WR. Continuous caudal analgesia. JAMA. 1943;123:538–46.
34. Martini J, Bacon DR, Vasdev GM. Edward Tuohy: the man, his needle, and its place in obstetric analgesia. RAPM. 2002;27:520–3.
35. Martinez Curbelo M. Anestesia peridural continua segmentaria con cateter ureteral utlizando la aguja de Tuohy caliber 16 con punta de Huber. Reunion Anual de Cirujanos Cubanos. La Havana, Enero 26. 1947.
36. Aldrete JA, Cabrera HS, Wright AJ. Manuel Martinez Curbelo and continuous lumbar epidural anesthesia. Bull Anesth Hist. 2004;22:4–8.
37. Flowers CE, Hellman LM, Hingson RA. Continuous peridural anesthesia and analgesia for labor, delivery and cesarean section. Curr Res Anesth Anal. 1949;28:181–9.
38. Bromage PR. Spinal epidural analgesia. London: Livingstone; 1954.

39. Bromage PR. Epidural analgesia. Philadelphia: Saunders; 1978.
40. Bonica JJ. Management of pain. Philadelphia: Lea & Febiger; 1953.
41. Bonica JJ, Backup PH, Anderson CE, Hasfield D, Crepps WF, Monk BF. Peridural block: analysis of 3,637 cases and a review. Anesthesiology. 1957;18:723–84.
42. Bonica JJ. Principles and practice of obstetric analgesia & anesthesia. Philadelphia: FA Davies; 1967.
43. Bonica JJ, McDonald JS. Principles and practice of obstetric analgesia & anesthesia. Philadelphia: Williams and Wilkins; 1995.

Anatomy of the Lumbar Epidural Region

Vertebral lumbar column anatomy and its attachments must be well known in order to have a mental picture of the course the needle should take during lumbar puncture.

The ligamentum flavum is one of the most important structures involved in epidural anesthesia. Its identification is essential to the loss of resistance technique (LORT) which relies on the distinctive resistance to needle advancement and fluid injection elicited by the ligamentum flavum. The very first small resistance encountered when the epidural needle is advanced in the lumbar region with a median approach is due to the density of the supraspinous ligament, followed by the feeling of no resistance when the needle is eventually advanced through the loose interspinous ligament. The knowledge of these two ligaments is therefore also crucial to performing the epidural technique.

The anatomy of the intervertebral foramen is important to understand the diffusion of the local anesthetic solutions in the epidural space, since it represents the doorway between the spinal canal and the periphery. Epidural fat distribution and epidural vein locations complete the essential basic background necessary to successfully carry out every epidural technique. The microscopic architecture of different tissue layers can help to better understand the mechanism of technical failures and complications.

2.1 Vertebral Column

The vertebral column is a curved linkage of individual bones or vertebrae. Its function is to support the trunk, to protect the spinal cord and nerves, and to provide attachments for the muscles.

A continuous series of vertebral foramina runs through the articulated vertebrae posterior to their bodies and constitutes the vertebral canal, inside which there is the dural sac containing the spinal cord and nerve roots, their coverings, and vasculature. A series of paired lateral intervertebral foramina permits communication between the lumen of the vertebral canal and the paravertebral soft tissues and accesses the passage of the spinal nerves and their associate vessels between adjacent vertebrae.

The adult vertebral column consists of 33 vertebral segments, each (except the first two cervical) separated from its neighbor by a fibrocartilaginous intervertebral disc. The usual number of the vertebrae is 7 cervical, 12 thoracic, 5 lumbar, 5 sacral, and 4 coccygeal for a total length of approximately 70 (male)–60 (female) cm. The fact that the vertebrae are separate units gives flexibility to the vertebral column. The joint between the bodies of two vertebrae is fibrocartilaginous, the union between the arches is ligamentous, and the joint between the articular processes is synovial in type.

G. Capogna, *Epidural Technique In Obstetric Anesthesia*,
https://doi.org/10.1007/978-3-030-45332-9_2

In adults, the vertebral column has four curvatures that change the cross-sectional profile of the trunk. The cervical curve is a lordosis (convex forward) and is the less marked. The thoracic curve is a kyphosis (convex dorsally) that extends from the second to the 11th–12th thoracic vertebrae; the lumbar curve is also a lordosis and has a greater magnitude in females and in pregnancy, and extends from the 12th thoracic to the lumbosacral angle. The pelvic curve is concave anteroinferiorly and involves the sacrum and the coccygeal vertebrae.

2.2　Lumbar Vertebra

The lumbar vertebra anatomy and its attachments should be well known in order to have a mental picture of the course the needle should take during lumbar puncture.

A typical vertebra is made up of a body, which bears weight and forms the base for the arch, composed of pedicles and laminae, which sur-

round and protect the cord laterally and posteriorly (Fig. 2.1). There are seven projections from these vertebral arches. There are three processes, two transverse and one spinous, for the attachment of muscles and ligaments, and four articular processes, two upper and two lower, to articulate with processes of the arches of the two neighboring vertebrae.

The five lumbar vertebrae are distinguished by their large size and absence of costal facets and transverse foramina. Their body is kidney shaped, wider transversally and deeper in front. The flat articular surface of the vertebral body is covered with hyaline cartilage which is very firmly united to the fibrocartilaginous intervertebral disc, this union being reinforced by anterior and posterior longitudinal ligamentous bands, which run the whole length of the vertebral column.

The pedicles are short and together with articular processes constitute the boundaries of the intervertebral foramen. The spinous process is almost horizontal, quadrangular, and thickened along its posterior and inferior borders. The trans-

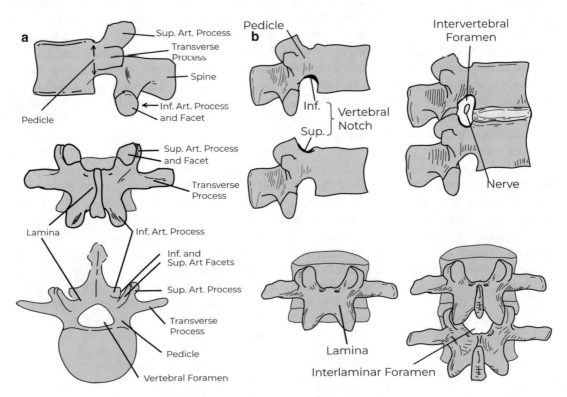

Fig. 2.1 (a, b) Anatomy of lumbar vertebra

verse processes are thin and long. The articular facets are reciprocally concave (superior) and convex (inferior) which allow flexion, extension, lateral bending, and some degree of rotation.

The interlaminar foramen is small and triangular in shape when the vertebral column is extended. The base is formed of the upper border of the laminae of the lower vertebra, and the sides of the medial aspects of the inferior articular processes of the vertebra above. During flexion the inferior articular process slides upwards and the interlaminar foramen enlarges and becomes diamond shaped, since the medial borders of the upper articular processes of the vertebra below now form the lower lateral boundaries of the aperture (Fig. 2.2). The interlaminar foramen is closed by the ligamenta flava.

2.3   Ligamentum Flavum

The ligamentum flavum is an important structure involved in epidural anesthesia. Its identification is essential to the loss of resistance technique (LORT) which relies on the distinctive resistance to needle advancement and fluid injection elicited by the ligamentum flavum.

It is rectangular/trapezoidal in shape, and is 13–20 mm high and 12–22 mm wide, and its thickness may vary from 3 to 5 mm [1] (Fig. 2.3).

The ligamentum flavum embryologically consists of a left and a right portion which usually fuse in the midline in the adult. The degree of midline fusion varies between individuals and across vertebral heights and midline gaps are more frequent in the cervical and high thoracic

Fig. 2.2 Dimension and shape of the interlaminar foramen when the vertebral column is extended or flexed

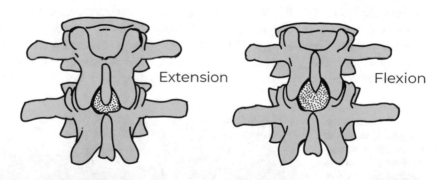

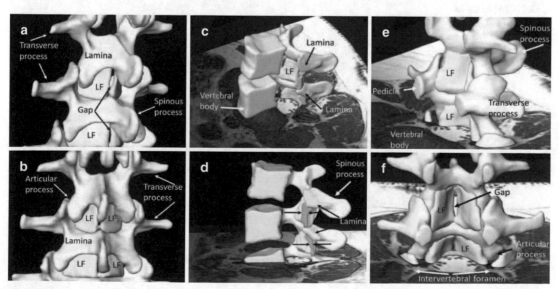

Fig. 2.3 3D reconstruction of human lumbar ligamentum flavum (LF). (**a**) Posterior-lateral view; (**b**) posterior view; (**c, d**) lateral view (sagittal section); (**e**) anterior lateral view; (**f**) anterior view (from [3] with permission)

regions. However ligamentum flavum midline gaps may also be present in approximately 20% of cases in the lumbar region too, especially between the L1 and L2 level [2] (Fig. 2.4).

Ligamenta flava connect laminae of adjacent vertebrae in the vertebral canal. They run from the anterior and inferior aspects of one lamina to the posterior and superior aspects of the lamina below. It laterally extends as far as the interlaminar foramen where it blends with the capsule of the articular processes. Here small foramina give passage to veins. Posteriorly they are bordered by the spinous muscles (multifidus) and in the midline the two ligamenta flava meet to become continuous with the deep fibers of the interspinous ligament. Anteriorly they are bordered by a mixture of fatty or loose connective tissue ("epidural space"). The upper border of the ligamenta flava of the same intervertebral space joins medially in an angle of more than 90° opening upwards. The internal surfaces form an angle of less than 90° opening towards the epidural space and a vertex merging with the interspinous ligament.

The topographical relationship of the ligamenta flava with the spinous, transverse, and articular processes and dural sac has recently been reviewed by using postmortem samples and magnetic resonance imaging in living humans [3]. In a 3D reconstruction, the ligamenta flava span from the external facet of the superior border of the caudal vertebrae to the inner facet of the inferior border of the cranial vertebrae. The inferior and lateral portion of the ligamentum makes contact with the paravertebral muscles. The medial border reaches the spinous process and the lateral border extends towards the intervertebral foramen and merges with the joint capsule of the articular facets. At the most lateral parts of the epidural space, where there is no epidural fat, the ligamenta flava directly contact the dural sac (Fig. 2.5a, b).

The predominant tissue is yellow elastic tissue ("flavus" is Latin for "yellow"), whose almost perpendicular fibers descend from the lower anterior surface of one lamina to the posterior surface and upper margin of the lamina below. This

Fig. 2.4 Anatomy of the paired ligamentum flavum spanning out between adjacent laminae (from Reina et al. (2015) Atlas of functional anatomy for regional anesthesia and pain medicine. Springer, with permission)

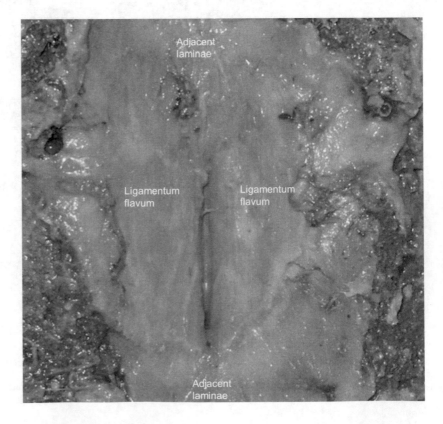

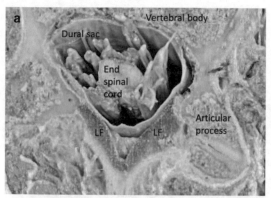

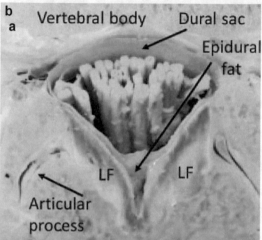

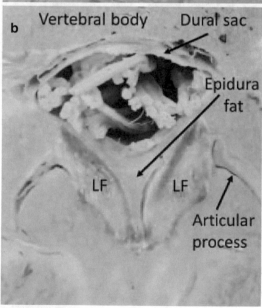

Fig. 2.5 (a) Transverse section of human lumbar spine at L1 vertebral level. *LF* ligamentum flavum (from [3] with permission). (**B**) Transverse section of human lumbar spine at L3 vertebral level (**a**, **b**). *LF* ligamentum flavum (from [3] with permission)

high content of elastic and elaunin fibers and the favorable proportion of elastic to collagen fibers (2:1) give this ligament elastic properties [4, 5].

The ligaments are thickest and strongest in the lumbar region since their role is to arrest separation of the laminae in spinal flexion, preventing abrupt limitation, and also to assist restoration to an erect posture after flexion, protecting the discs from injury. When the spine is flexed the ligamentum flavum is stretched and stores mechanical energy, which is regained upon extension of the spinal column. Fine free fiber nerve endings innervate the outermost layer of this ligament, most likely related to positional control.

The thickness of the ligamentum may vary with vertebral level, body mass index, disc herniation, and age [6]. In addition it is not uniform even within the single intervertebral space, and most likely its thickness may also decrease if the back is well flexed and the ligament very stretched. Finally the method of assessment of its thickness (cadaveric studies, magnetic resonance, computed tomography, or ultrasound studies in living subjects) may also affect the precise measurement [7].

2.4   Interspinous and Supraspinous Ligaments

The very first small resistance encountered when the epidural needle is advanced in the lumbar region with a median approach is due to the density of the supraspinous ligament, followed by the feeling of no resistance when the needle is eventually advanced through the loose interspinous ligament.

Interspinous ligaments are thin, almost membranous and connect adjoining spines, since their attachments extend from the root to the apex of each. They meet the ligamenta flava in front and the supraspinous ligament behind. These ligaments are thick and quadrilateral at lumbar levels. Their ventral part may be regarded as a posterior extension of the ligamentum flavum and contains a few elastic fibers. The middle part is the main component and is purely collagenous. The dorsal part is also collagenous and its fibers continue with the supraspinous ligament and the medial tendons of the multifidus muscle.

The supraspinous ligament is commonly described as a strong fibrous cord which connects the tips of the spinous process from C7 to the sacrum, and it is thicker and broader at lumbar levels (Fig. 2.6).

However, there is evidence to support the definition of supraspinous and interspinous ligaments as structures formed of a combination of muscle tendons and aponeuroses along the length of the thoracic and lumbar spine, with regional differ-

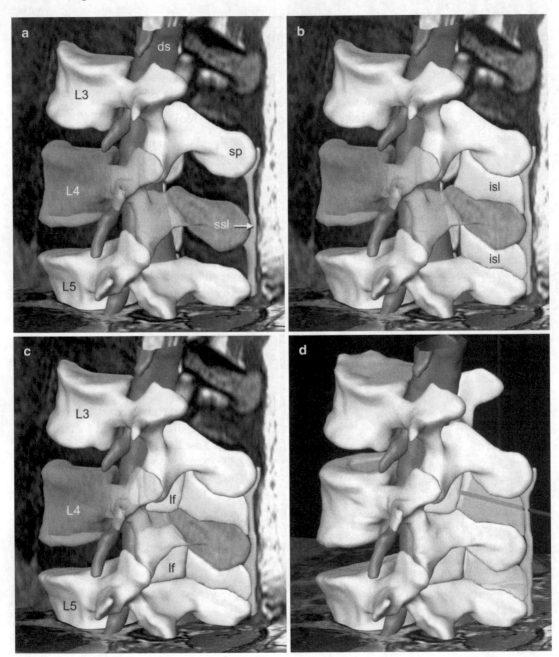

Fig. 2.6 Posterior ligaments of interest in lumbar epidural block. Supraspinous ligament (ssl), spinous process (sp), interspinous ligament (isl), ligamentum flavum (lf), dural sac (ds). 3D models built from axial (**a–d**) and sagit-tal (**a–c**) T2-weighted reference images (from Reina et al. (2015) Atlas of functional anatomy for regional anesthesia and pain medicine. Springer, with permission)

Fig. 2.7 (**a**) Formation of the lumbar supraspinous ligament by trapezius (trap-double arrows) and the posterior layer of thoracolumbar fascia (single arrowheads) orientated in the rostral (r) to caudal (c) direction. (**b**) Horizontal slice at L3 level. Formation of the supraspinous ligament by the posterior layer of the thoracolumbar fascia. Longissimus thoracis (lt) and multifidus (m) attached to the spinous process (sp) laterally. (**c**) Horizontal slice at L1–L2 level. The contribution of the posterior layer of the thoracolumbar fascia, multifidus, and longissimus thoracis to the interspinous ligament. The interspinous ligament merges with the ligamentum flavum (lf) and capsule of the zygapophyseal joint (za) (bar scales = 4 mm) (from [8] with permission)

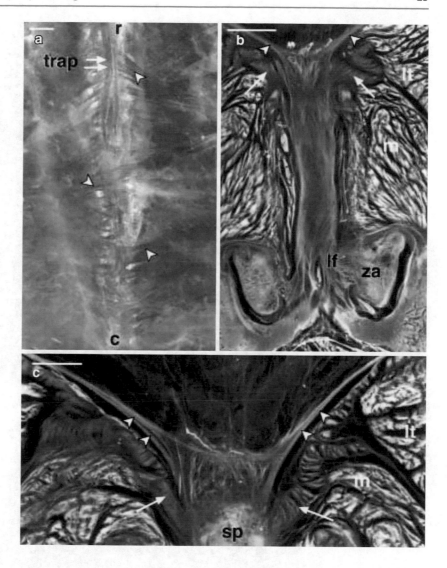

ences in their connective structure [8] (Figs. 2.7 and 2.8).

The midline attachments of the posterior layer of the thoracolumbar fascia and the longissimus thoracis with the contribution of the fascia of the muscle multifidus form the main dense connective tissue component of both the supraspinous and interspinous ligaments at the lumbar level.

While in the thoracic area no interspinous ligament is detectable, at lumbar level, where the posterior layer of the thoracolumbar fascia joins the other tendinous insertion, the interspinous ligament becomes recognizable as a separate anatomical entity.

Wide variation in fiber direction in the connective tissue architecture within both the interspinous and supraspinous ligaments can be explained together with their biomechanical function to limit flexion. The multiple directions of connective tissue fibers within the ligaments indicate that they are capable of transmitting loads in more than one direction.

Since they both originate from the same connective tissues (thoracolumbar fascia, longissimus thoracis, and multifidus fascia) it may be considered difficult, at the lumbar level, to consider the supraspinous and interspinous ligaments as a separate entity. The average depth of

Fig. 2.8 (**a**) Horizontal slice at L3 level. Connective tissue fiber orientation within the supraspinous ligament and attachments to the spinous process (sp). Anteriorly (single-dashed arrow), obliquely (double-dashed arrows), and horizontally (triple-dashed arrows) directed fibers are evident. The posterior layer of the thoracolumbar fascia (single arrowheads) and shared attachment (single arrow) from longissimus thoracis (lt) and multifidus (m). (**b**) Horizontal slice at L5 level. Decussation of connective tissue fibers (double arrowheads) from the posterior layer of the thoracolumbar fascia is visible superficial to the erector spinae aponeuroses. Multifidus merges with the interspinous ligament to attach onto the spinous process (bar scales – 4 mm) (from [8] with permission)

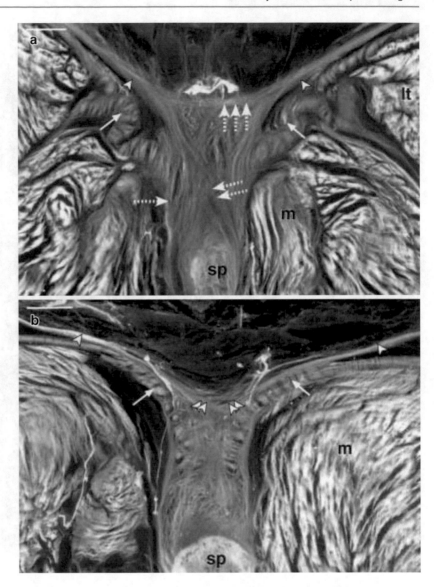

the supraspinous-interspinous complex ranges, in the young female, between 24 and 30 mm [9].

2.5 Muscles

In the case of the epidural paramedian approach technique, the needle avoids the supraspinous and interspinous ligaments, and reaches the ligamentum flavum penetrating the paraspinous muscles: erector spinae and multifidus.

The erector spinae (sacrospinalis) lies on either side of the vertebral column. It forms a large musculotendinous mass which varies in size and composition at different levels. At the lumbar and sacral levels it narrows and becomes tendinous as it approaches its attachments. In the upper lumbar region it expands to form three columns (iliocostalis, longissimus, and spinalis). It arises from the anterior surface of a large aponeurosis which is attached to the median and lateral sacral crest and the spines of the lumbar and the

11th and 12th thoracic vertebrae with their supraspinous ligaments. This muscle has numerous functions, such as back extension, lateral back flexion, and rotation.

The multifidus muscle is a multipennate muscle and is the most medial paraspinal muscle lying lateral to the spinous process [10]. Its fibers are continuous with the erector spinae and its aponeurosis contributes to the formation of the interspinous and supraspinous ligaments (Fig. 2.8). Its function is to stabilize the lumbar spine in the transverse plane.

2.6 Intervertebral Foramen and Its Ligaments

Knowledge of the anatomy of the intervertebral foramen is important to understand the diffusion of the local anesthetic solutions in the epidural space, since it represents the doorway between the spinal canal and the periphery. The boundaries of this foramen consist of two movable joints, the ventral intervertebral joint and the dorsal zygapophysial joint, and it is essentially a large osseous hole though which structures pass. The intervertebral foramen transmits the spinal nerves, spinal arteries and veins, recurrent meningeal nerves, and lymphatics. The intervertebral foramen has ligaments crossing its openings and their morphology may vary from L1 to L5. They serve a protective and organizational role for the neurovascular structures of the foramen [11, 12]. They may be designated into internal, intraforaminal, and external ligaments and their arrangement causes the intervertebral foramen to be partitioned into smaller compartments for the passage of the spinal artery, for the ventral ramus of the spinal nerve, for the recurrent meningeal nerve and the segmental artery, and for the passage of the dorsal ramus of the spinal nerve and its accompanying vessels, and a compartment for the veins (Fig. 2.9).

Epidural fat surrounds each nerve root throughout their course to the intervertebral fora-

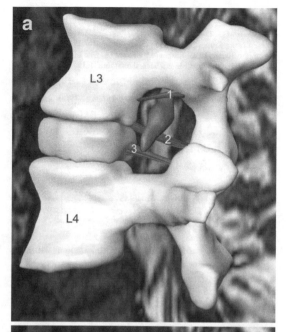

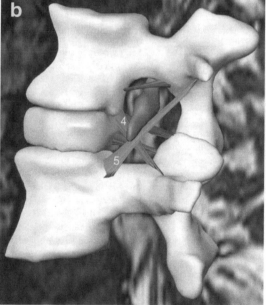

Fig. 2.9 The main transforaminal ligaments (a group of collagen condensations that compartmentalize the intervertebral foramen). (**a**) Deep and middle layers: (1) oblique superior, (2) mid-transforaminal, and (3) oblique inferior. (**b**) Superficial layers: (4) superior corporotransverse and (5) inferior corporo-transverse (from Reina et al. (2015) Atlas of functional anatomy for regional anesthesia and pain medicine. Springer, with permission)

men. The nerve roots, once located in the inter-vertebral foramen, commonly combine to form the spinal nerve. Just prior to the formation of the spinal nerve a small enlargement of the dorsal root is noted. This enlargement is called the dorsal root ganglion (DRG) which contains the cell bodies of sensory neurons. At lumbar level the DRG is located within the anatomic boundaries of the intervertebral foramen, usually directly beneath the foramen.

2.7 Epidural Space

Immediately outside the epidural mater there is the epidural space which extends from the foramen magnum to the sacral hiatus. The epidural space is in part real, filled with adipose tissue, nerve roots, veins, arteries, and lymphatics, and in part virtual, with the dural sac resting on the vertebral bodies, pedicles, laminae, and ligamentum flavum [13, 14].

2.7.1 Epidural Fat

Epidural fat is the main component of the epidural space, contributes to its shape, has a metameric and a discontinuous topography, and is mainly located in the posterior and in the lateral region, around the nerve cuffs (Fig. 2.10). Nerve cuffs are lateral prolongations of the dura mater, arachnoid lamina, and pia mater that enclose nerve roots in their way across the epidural space towards the intervertebral foramen, and the dorsal root ganglion, located within the intervertebral foramen.

Epidural fat is relatively metabolically inactive and it is not a simple space-filling tissue. Fascicles of connective tissue are less numerous and thinner than in subcutaneous fat with

Fig. 2.10 3D reconstruction of human epidural fat. Posterior (**a**) and lateral (**b**) view (from Reina et al. (2015) Atlas of functional anatomy for regional anesthesia and pain medicine. Springer, with permission)

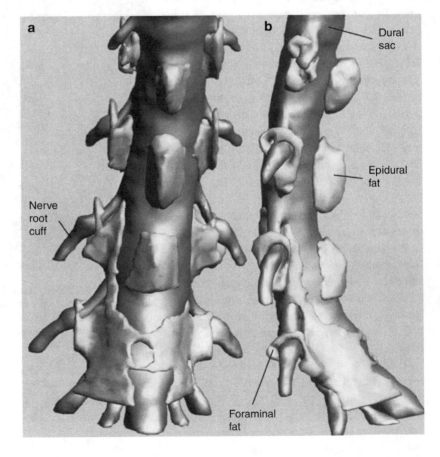

organized sliding spaces (Fig. 2.11). These slits are unique to epidural fat [15]. This histological feature, together with the fact that rarely adheres to the bony structures, suggests that posterior epidural fat plays the role of a sliding structure between the posterior surface of the dural sac and the anterior surface of the vertebral arch, protecting the dural sac and its components against the effects of lashing, deceleration, and rotational forces due to vertebral column movements. Therefore, posterior epidural fat appears to be a functional part of the spinal unit. Epidural fat is also commonly believed to act as a storage place for lipophilic drugs injected into the epidural space, but little is known as to how it can influence the kinetics of injected solutions.

Epidural fat has different distributions in the cervical, thoracic, lumbar, and sacral levels and this distribution remains constant along each vertebral level. At the cervical level it is almost absent; in the thoracic region it forms a broad posterior band thicker near the intervertebral disc. At lumbar levels the epidural fat forms two separate, unconnected structures anteriorly and laterally (lateral and foraminal fat). At the sacral level posterior epidural fat gets its greatest volume (Fig. 2.12).

The epidural fat extends cranio-caudally from the inferior aspect of one vertebral lamina to the superior aspect of the lamina of the sub-adjacent vertebra and in the lateral direction towards the point where the articular facets and ligamentum flavum intersect (posterior epidural space). It also fills the space between the vertebral arches and intervertebral foramina wrapping the nerve root cuffs (lateral epidural space).

At the lumbar level the volume of posterior epidural fat increases caudally from L1-2 to L4-5. The average height of this fat is 16–25 mm and the width increases cranio-caudally from 6 to 13 mm [16].

The anterior epidural space may be considered as a separate compartment, defined by fibrous connective bands (ligaments of Hofmann) which are firmly connected to the posterior longitudinal ligament and that anchor it anteriorly to the posterior surface of the vertebral body. The arrangement of such ligaments suggests their supportive and protective role in stabilizing and anchoring the dural sac and by that, the spinal cord and spinal nerves, to the bony vertebral canal [17].

The presence of such a ligament defines two medial cavities which enclose anterior and medial venous plexuses (which together receive the basivertebral veins) and two lateral cavities which receive the anterior longitudinal veins. Contents of the medial and lateral cavities pass freely between the two. The lateral cavity con-

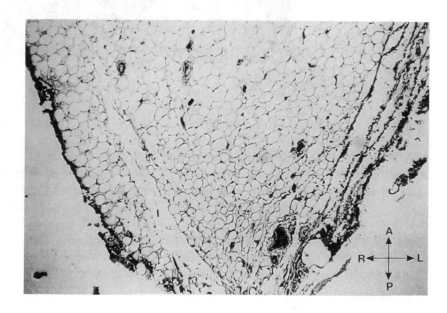

Fig. 2.11 Axial section of posterior epidural fat (×680). Adipocytes are homogeneous in size and shape and connective tissue is scarce. In subcutaneous fat instead, size and shape of adipocytes are variable and connective tissue is sizeable. *A* anterior side close to the dural sac, *P* posterior side, *R* right side close to the right ligamenta flava, *L* left side close to the left ligamenta flava (from [15] with permission)

Fig. 2.12 3D reconstruction of human epidural fat. Lateral (**a**), anterior (**b**), and oblique (**c**) view of epidural fat among vertebrae. Anterior (**d**) complete view of epidural fat without vertebrae (from Reina et al. (2015) Atlas of functional anatomy for regional anesthesia and pain medicine. Springer, with permission)

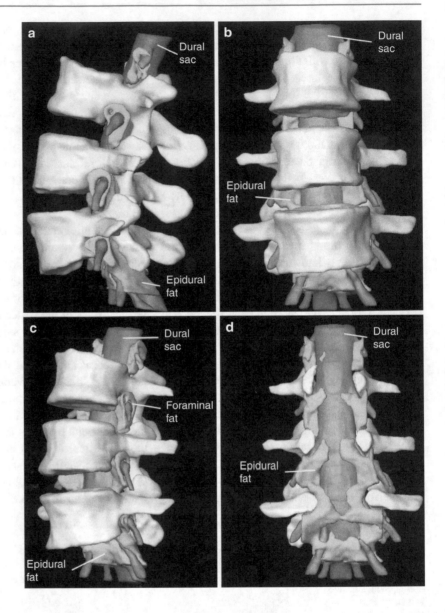

nects to the intervertebral canal and dorsally into the posterior epidural space [18].

The satisfactoriness of epidural anesthesia may not be affected by the anatomical arrangement of the dorsal epidural ligaments since the primary target of the anesthetic agents in the epidural space is the nerve cuffs.

Structures which are contained in the epidural space and that pass through the spinal foramina include the nerve root cuffs, lymphatic vessels, spinal branch of the segmental artery, and communicating veins between the internal and external vertebral venous plexuses. All these structures are surrounded by adipose tissue and fibrous ligaments attaching nerve root cuffs to the bones. At the lumbar levels the craniocaudal diameter of the intervertebral foramen is between 19–21 mm and the anteroposterior diameter varies from 9–11 mm (superiorly) to 7–9 mm (inferiorly).

At this level the spinal nerve is located in the upper third of the foramen and size of the nerve root within the nerve root cuffs has a diameter of 5–6 mm up to 10–12 mm around the ganglion [19].

2.7.2 Nerve Roots and Nerve Root Cuff

Nerve rootlets leave the spinal cord at the antero-lateral and posterolateral sulci. They are most numerous at lumbar level, and join to form the anterior roots (from the 6–8 anterior rootlets) and the posterior roots (from the 8–10 posterior rootlets). Anterior (ventral) roots contain mostly efferent fibers from anterior and lateral spinal gray columns. At thoracic and lumbar levels they also carry pre-

ganglionic sympathetic fibers from the lateral horn. Posterior (dorsal) roots contain centripetal processes of neurons sited in the dorsal root ganglia. Inside the epidural space, spinal nerve roots are enclosed by lateral prolongation of dura mater and arachnoideal lamina: the dural cuff. Spinal nerve cuff microscopic morphology resembles that of the spinal subdural compartment in the dural sac, suggesting the possibility of a transitional leptomeningeal cellular structure shared also with neurothelial cells from the subdural compartment, arachnoid, and pia cells. Not only the lateral epidural fat around the spinal nerve cuff, but also the fat (adipocytes) located inside the cuff, next to the axons, could influence the absorption and distribution of drugs injected in the epidural space [20] (Fig. 2.13).

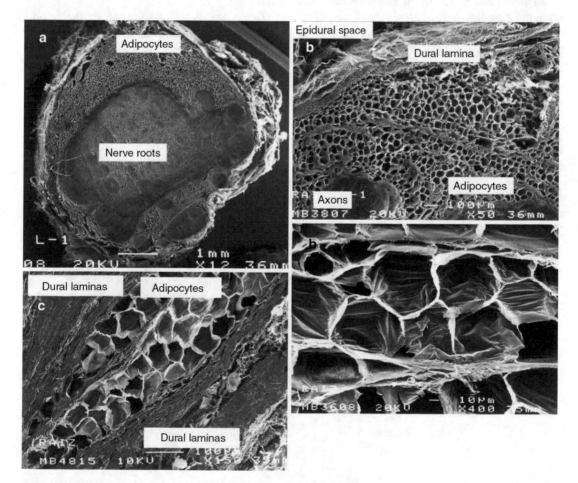

Fig. 2.13 Spinal nerve root cuff. (**a**) Complete view of a nerve root cuff (transversal cut). (**b**, **c**) Dural laminas and adipocytes. (**d**) Sample shows adipocytes cut in halves. Scanning electron microscopy (×12–×400) (from [20] with permission)

2.7.3 Internal Vertebral Venous Plexus, Epidural Arteries, and Lymphatics

Intervertebral veins accompany the spinal nerves through the intervertebral foramen and drain blood from the internal vertebral plexus which is located inside the epidural space (Fig. 2.14). The internal vertebral venous plexus, also known as the epidural venous plexus or as Batson's plexus, is located mainly in the anterior aspect of the epidural space.

This venous plexus, which drains blood not only from the cord but also from the vertebral bodies via large basivertebral veins, consists of several anterior and posterior longitudinal and interconnecting vessels.

At the lumbar level the posterior vertebral veins seem to be rudimentary or poorly developed [21].

The veins of the internal vertebral venous plexus contain no valves; therefore the direction of drainage is posture and respiration dependent.

The internal vertebral venous plexus provides an alternate route of venous return when the jugular veins of the neck are compressed, when the flow through the inferior vena cava is obstructed, and when intrathoracic or intra-abdominal pressures are increased.

Obstruction of the inferior vena cava such as in pregnancy diverts a proportion of the venous return from the legs and pelvic structure into the vertebral venous system, which is composed of three freely communicating valveless networks: intraosseous vertebral veins, paravertebral veins, and epidural venous plexus. Of these, the engorged epidural venous plexus is expected to decrease the effective capacity of the epidural and subarachnoid spaces. These decreased spaces are considered to be one of the reasons for the pregnancy-induced enhancement of regional anesthesia.

The epidural arteries located in the lumbar region of the vertebral column are branches of the iliolumbar arteries. These arteries are found in the lateral region of the space and therefore are not usually threatened by an advancing epidural needle.

Fig. 2.14 Vertebral and epidural venous system

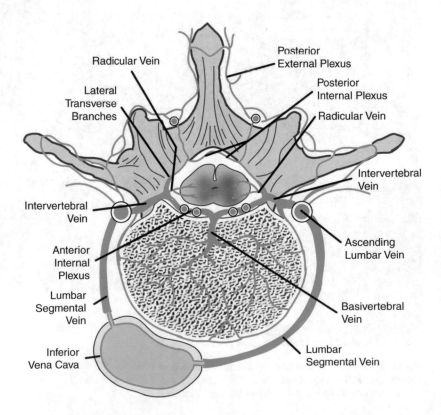

The lymphatics of the epidural space are concentrated in the region of the dural roots where they remove foreign materials including microorganisms from the subarachnoid and epidural spaces.

2.8   Dural Sac

The dural sac surrounds the spinal cord inside the vertebral column. It separates the epidural space from the subarachnoid space, ending at the second sacral vertebra (Fig. 2.15). The dura mater is the most external layer of the dural sac and is responsible for 90% of its total thickness. This fibrous structure provides mechanical protection to the spinal cord and its neural elements. The internal 10% of the dural sac is formed by the arachnoid layer, which is a cellular lamina that adds little extra mechanical resistance. In the lumbar region, the dural sac is, on the average, 0.3 mm thick.

2.8.1   Dura Mater

The spinal dura mater is the outermost meningeal membrane enclosing the spinal cord. It is attached to the circumference of the foramen magnum, and the posterior surface of the bodies of the second and third cervical vertebrae. At the level of the second sacral vertebra it invests the filum terminale and descends to the posterior aspect of the coccyx, where it blends with the periosteum.

At the spinal level the dura mater is composed of collagen fibers, 0.1 μm thick, oriented in different directions and of approximately 80 concentric laminas, each approximately 5 μm thick, formed of thinner laminas (subunits) containing mostly collagen fibers (Fig. 2.16). The collagen fibers do not traverse different dural lamina. The collagen fibers are oriented in different directions but always within the concentric plane of the dural lamina. The elastic fibers are fewer, measuring 2 μm in diameter, and have a rougher surface than that of the collagen fibers [22].

2.8.2   Arachnoid Layer

In the past the arachnoid membrane was defined as a fine layer in contact but not adhering to the internal surface of the dura mater separated by the so-called subdural space. This concept has now been modified [23]. The arachnoid layer

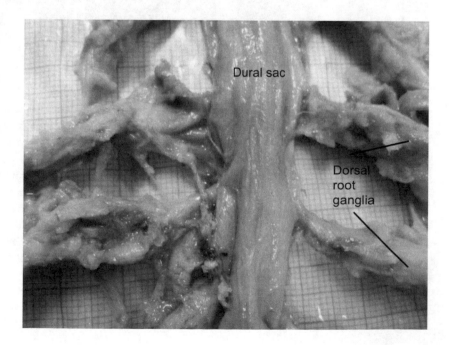

Fig. 2.15 Human dural sac and nerve root cuffs. Posterior surface at lumbar level (from Reina et al. (2015) Atlas of functional anatomy for regional anesthesia and pain medicine. Springer, with permission)

Dural sac

Dorsal root ganglia

Fig. 2.16 Human dura mater. (**a**) Full thickness (magnification ×300). (**b**) Detail of thickness of four dural laminas (magnification ×4000) (from Reina et al. (2015) Atlas of functional anatomy for regional anesthesia and pain medicine. Springer, with permission)

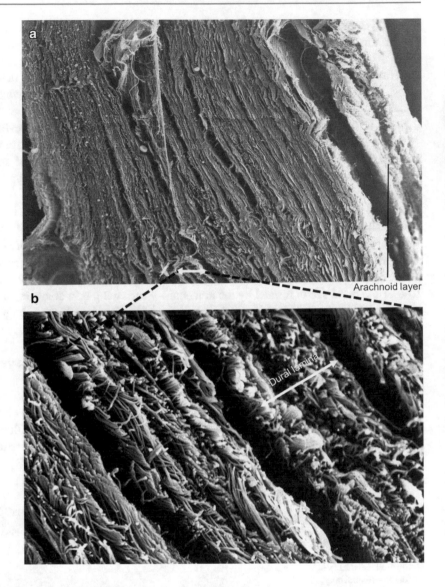

Arachnoid layer

Dural lamina

(Fig. 2.17) is a semipermeable membrane which exerts a barrier against the substances across it. It is about 30–40 μm thick and is composed by cells strongly bonded by a specific membrane junction. Four well-differentiated structures can be observed from the outer towards the inner aspect of the membrane: (a) the outermost area constituted by neurothelial cells (dural border or subdural compartment); (b) collagen fibers which occupy approximately 40–50% of the total thickness; (c) the arachnoid cell layer, constituted by four or five cellular planes joined together by tight junctions and limited by a basal membrane, which limits the passage of substances;

and (d) the innermost area which lies in direct contact with the cerebrospinal fluid and which is formed of reticular or trabecular arachnoid. This layer gives shape to tubular structures (arachnoid sheaths) for each nerve root and for the spinal cord (Fig. 2.18). This arachnoid network limits nerve root movement to a certain extent, holding each root in its position within the dural sac. These sheaths may be responsible for the partial or total failure of spinal anesthesia should the spinal needle inadvertently enters the sheaths and deposits the local anesthetic solution inside them. In this case the local anesthetic solution can diffuse in an anomalous or incomplete way, following a single

Fig. 2.17 Dissection of dural sac at the level of cauda equina. The arachnoid membrane appears as a translucent membrane (from [24] with permission)

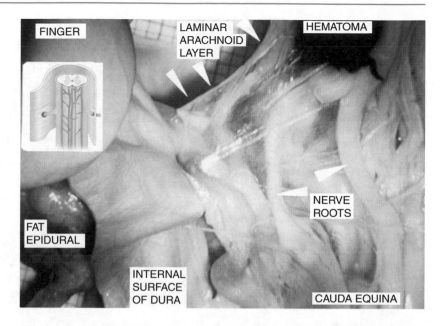

Fig. 2.18 Trabecular arachnoid. Detail of four spinal nerve roots with their arachnoid sheaths. Scanning electron microscopy. Magnification ×100 (from Reina et al. (2015) Atlas of functional anatomy for regional anesthesia and pain medicine. Springer, with permission)

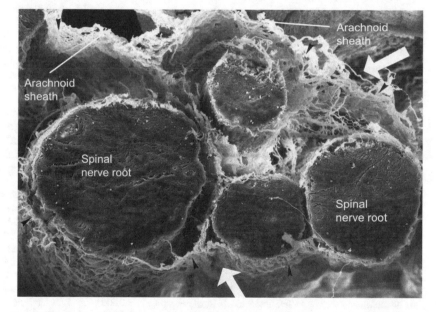

nerve root rather than spreading uniformly to all the roots contained in the dural sac.

2.8.3   Subdural and Intradural Space

Ultrastructural studies have demonstrated that there is no space between the dura and the arachnoid [24]. Between the last dural lamina and the arachnoid layer there is a tissue com-posed of neurothelial cells surrounded by an amorphous substance (Fig. 2.19). This thin layer is susceptible to tearing and the low cohesion forces between neurothelial cells may facilitate the widening of a minimal fissure to yield a subdural space. Therefore the so-called subdural space is not a potential space as previously thought, but is only produced as a result of trauma and tissue damage creating a cleft within the meninges.

Fig. 2.19 Dura-arachnoid interface seen below the dural lamina (most internal aspect of the dura). The dura-arachnoid interface is filled with neurothelial cells and amorphous material. Transmission electron microscopy, magnification ×5000 (from [24] with permission)

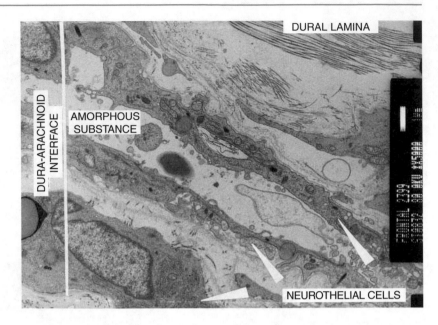

The intradural space is also an artifactual space [25], concentric and parallel to the dural layers, that may be produced, accidentally and in certain conditions, by needle or catheter insertion and may be formed by dural delamination rather than by its tearing.

References

1. Zarzur E. Anatomic studies of the human lumbar ligamentum flavum. Anesth Analg. 1984;63:499–502.
2. Lirk P, Moriggl B, Colvin J, et al. The incidence of lumbar ligamentum flavum midline gaps. Anesth Analg. 2004;98:1178–80.
3. Reina M, Lirk P, Sàncez AP, et al. Human lumbar ligamentum flavum anatomy for epidural anesthesia. Reviewing a 3D MR-based interactive model and postmortem samples. Anesth Analg. 2016;122:903–7.
4. Nachemson AL, Evans JH. Some mechanical properties of the third human lumbar interlaminar ligament (ligamentum flavum). J Biomech. 1968;3:211–4.
5. Yahia LH, Garzon S, Strykowski H, et al. Ultrastructure of the human interspinous ligament and ligamentum flavum. A preliminary study. Spine. 1990;15:262–8.
6. Altinkaia N, Yldirim T, Demir S, et al. Factors associated with the thickness of the ligamentum flavum: is ligamentum flavum thickening due to hypertrophy or buckling? Spine. 2011;36(16):E1093–7.
7. Kolte VS, Kambatta S, Ambiye MV. Thickness of the ligamentum flavum: correlation with age and its asymmetry. A magnetic resonance imaging study. Asian Spine J. 2014;9:245–53.
8. Johnson GM, Zhang M. Regional differences within the human supraspinous and interspinous ligaments: a sheet plastination study. Eur Spine J. 2002;11:382–8.
9. Jang D, Seoungwoo P. A morphometric study of the lumbar interspinous space in 100 Stanford University Medical Center patients. J Korean Neurosurg Soc. 2014;55:2661–266.
10. Lonneman ME, Paris SV, Gorniak GC. A morphological comparison of the human lumbar multifidus by chemical dissection. J Man Manip Ther. 2013;16(4):E84–92. https://doi.org/10.1179/jmt2008.16.4.84E.
11. Amonoo-Kuofi HA, El-Badawi M, Fatani J. Ligaments associated with lumbar intervertebral foramina. L1 to L4. J Anat. 1988;156:177–83.
12. Amonoo-Kuofi HA, El-Badawi M, Fatani J, et al. Ligaments associated with lumbar intervertebral foramina. The fifth lumbar level. J Anat. 1988;159:1–10.
13. Reina MA, Franco CD, Lòpez A, et al. Clinical implications of epidural fat in the spinal canal. A scanning electron microscopic study. Acta Anaesthesiol Belg. 2009;60:7–17.
14. Reina MA, Pulido P, Casteldo J, et al. Characteristics and distribution of normal human epidural fat. Rev Esp Anestesiol Reanim. 2006;53:363–72. (in Spanish).
15. Beaujeux R, Wolfram-Gabel R, Kehrli P, et al. Posterior lumbar epidural fat as a functional structure? Spine. 1997;22:1264–9.
16. Wolfram-Gabel R, Beaujeux R, Fabre M, et al. Histologic characteristics of posterior lumbar epidural fatty tissue. J Neuroradiol. 1996;23:19–25.
17. Wiltse L, Fonseca A, Amster J, et al. Relationship of the dura, Hofmann's ligaments, Baston's plexus

and a fibrovascular membrane lying on the posterior surface of the vertebral bodies and attaching to the deep layer of the posterior longitudinal ligament: an anatomical, radiologic and clinical study. Spine. 1993;18:1030–43.

18. Plaisant O, Sarrazin JL, Cosnard G, et al. The lumbar anterior epidural cavity: the posterior longitudinal ligament, the anterior ligaments of the dura mater and the anterior internal vertebral plexus. Acta Anat. 1996;155:274–81.

19. De Andrès J, Reina MA, Macès F, et al. Epidural fat: considerations for minimally invasive spinal injection and surgical therapies. JNR. 2011;1:45–53.

20. Reina MA, Villanueva MC, Machès F et al. The ultrastructure of the human spinal nerve root cuff in the lumbar spine. Anesth Analg. 2008;106:339–44.

21. Gerhater R, St Louis EL. Lumbar epidural venography: review of 1200 case. Neuroradiology. 1979;131:409–21.

22. Reina MA, Dittmann M, López A, et al. New perspectives in the microscopic structure of human dura mater in the dorso lumbar region. Reg Anesth. 2001;22:161–6.

23. Reina MA, Prats-Galino A, Sola RG, et al. Structure of the arachnoid layer of the human spinal meninges: a barrier that regulates dural sac permeability. Rev Esp Anestesiol Reanim. 2010;57:486–92.

24. Reina MA, De Leon Casasola O, Lòpez A, et al. The origin of the spinal subdural space: ultrastructure findings. Anesth Analg. 2002;94:991–5.

25. Collier CB, Reina MA, Prats-Galino A, et al. An anatomical study of the intradural space. Anaesth Intensive Care. 2011;39:1038–42.

Distribution of a Solution in the Epidural Space

"A number of variables determine how far neural blockade will spread after injection of an analgesic solution into the epidural space. Some of these are intrinsic to the patient, and some are extrinsic, depending on variations of technique and the drugs employed": with these words Philip Bromage opened his cornerstone paper *"Spread of analgesic solutions in the epidural space and their site of action"* in 1962 [1]. In this classical work he postulated that the spread from an epidural injection could have two components: (1) spread within the epidural space itself, depending on the volume, speed of injection, posture, age, height, etc., and (2) subdural and subpial spread, which could have been proportional to the diffusion coefficient, the area of contact, the concentration gradient, and the time of contact. He observed that ultimately the segmental spread was dependent on the mass of analgesic solute available for transneuronal diffusion in the epidural space. He also observed that the "appropriate mass of solute can be presented in the form of a large volume of weak solution, in which case it will travel widely in the epidural space and diffuse relatively poorly or as a very small volume of concentrated material … where presumably epidural spread was limited by the small volumes used, but where the neuraxial spread was extensive owing to the high concentration gradient." The final conclusions of Prof Bromage are still valid today: "The outcome of an epidural injection is the resultant of many different forces. If any of these is unusually weak, or another particularly strong, we may expect that clinical results will deviate from normal, and the accuracy of our results will depend on our ability to choose the appropriate dose with intelligent anticipation."

3.1 Sites of Action, Dynamics of Nerve Block, and Physicochemical Properties of Local Anesthetics

The spinal nerve roots are suggested to be the primary sites of action of epidural anesthesia [2, 3] although epidurally administered drugs may also eventually reach the spinal cord, crossing through the meninges and the spinal nerve root sleeves and diffusing into radicular arteries with subsequent transport to the spinal cord (even if the latter two mechanisms have been questioned) [4].

The spinal meninges are the main barrier to drug diffusion, the arachnoid mater accounting for nearly 90% of the resistance to diffusion through the meninges. The pia mater, with its tight cellular junctions, also presents an obstacle.

The earliest and widest local anesthetic contact with the nerve fibers is exactly where the spinal roots traverse the epidural space, extending to as far as the interlaminar foramina.

Along this tract the membranes covering the newly emergent nerve are least robust and may favor the local anesthetic penetration.

© Springer Nature Switzerland AG 2020
G. Capogna, *Epidural Technique In Obstetric Anesthesia*,
https://doi.org/10.1007/978-3-030-45332-9_3

The spinal nerve root size may also contribute to determine the degree of local anesthetic penetration and thus influence the anesthetic efficacy. Dorsal nerve roots are larger than the ventral roots [3]. Although a larger dorsal nerve root would seem more impenetrable to local anesthetics, the separation of the dorsal root into component bundles creates a much larger surface area for local anesthetic penetration than the single smaller ventral nerve root (Fig. 3.1). This anatomical finding may help to explain the relative ease of sensory versus motor block observed with the epidural block.

Once inside the nerve cuff, the local anesthetic must diffuse and penetrate through a multitude of tissue barriers. The perineurium, including fasciculi of hundreds of closely packed individual axons, is the greatest local anesthetic diffusion obstacle, because of tight cellular junctions in its innermost perilemma. Once through the nerve sheath, the intraneural local anesthetic solution front advances inwards radially from the exterior mantle to the core of the nerve. Motor efferent fibers, because of their longer internodal interval, are blocked later and their block lasts less than that of the pain conduction afferents.

The extraneural local anesthetic pool eventually decreases by dispersion, dilution, tissue binding, and absorption, and therefore, following a steady-state period, the diffusion gradient reverses outwards from the core to the mantle of the axon.

The physicochemical properties of local anesthetics, such as the degree of ionization and lipid solubility, may influence the extent of drug distribution in the axonal membrane, and may explain the differences in potency, onset time, and duration of anesthesia among local anesthetics [5, 6].

Potency has been shown to be related to lipid solubility [7] but this relationship may be complex, because high lipid solubility enhances the diffusion of the drug into membranes, but may become rate limited when a large fraction of the local anesthetic is in the ionized state. Moreover, the faster diffusion rate of the lipid-soluble drug can be counteracted by the capacity of the membrane to contain the drug in its lipophilic environment [8]. In addition to a greater lipid solubility, the longer acting local anesthetics show extensive protein binding. Both factors can contribute to a slower final nerve penetration rate. An increase in the degree of protein binding is thought to increase the duration of local anesthetic activity. Therefore, agents that penetrate the axolemma and attach more firmly to membrane proteins have a prolonged duration of anesthetic activity [9].

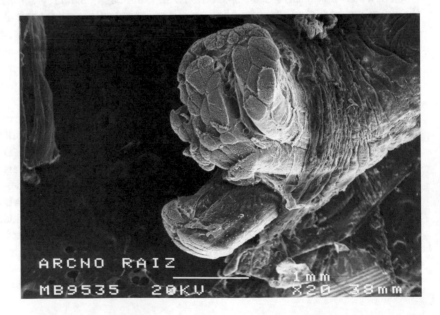

Fig. 3.1 Dorsal and ventral nerve roots (courtesy of Prof Miguel Angel Reina)

3.2   Local Tissue Distribution

From the epidural space drugs may go four ways: (1) exit the intervertebral foramina to reach the paravertebral area, (2) diffuse into ligaments, (3) diffuse across the spinal meninges and into the cerebrospinal fluid (CSF), and (4) distribute into epidural fat. The last two ways are the most important for the pharmacological effect.

Local anesthetics reach the spinal roots and the spinal cord from the cerebrospinal fluid (CSF) by passive diffusion [10].

Arachnoid villi, considered in the past as potential regions for drug transfer from the epidural space to the CSF and finally to the spinal cord, have been demonstrated to not contribute to opioid and local anesthetic diffusion across the meninges [11].

The nerve blocking effects of local anesthetics are counteracted by the uptake of the local anesthetics in epidural fat and vascular structures [12], especially the spinal radicular arteries that enhance their vascular removal [13]. Uptake in the epidural fat lowers the perineural concentration and thus reduces the clinical potency of the local anesthetic injected (Fig. 3.2). Additionally, it may prolong the duration of block, by providing a depot from which the local anesthetic dissociates slowly, maintaining a clinically significant perineural concentration [8, 14]. The area of the intervertebral foramina and the connective tissue surrounding the dural sleeves contain substantial amounts of fat. Drugs contained in the fat around the dural sleeves may have a greater influence on the nerve roots than drugs from the epidural fat, because of the higher concentrations and the shorter distance between the fat and the nerve roots [14]. However, this area is also found to be highly vascularized [15] favoring the systemic uptake of local anesthetic.

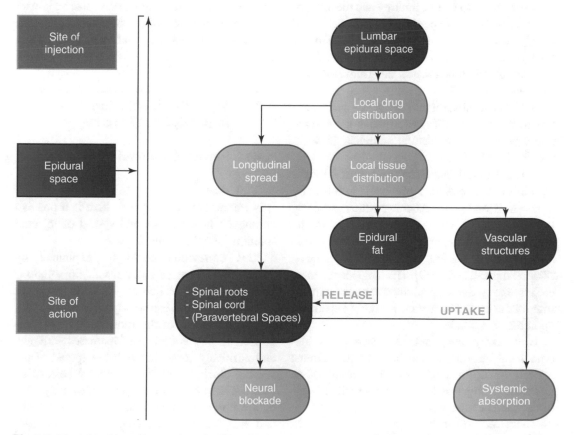

Fig. 3.2 Nerve blocking effects and uptake of local anesthetics in the epidural space

In conclusion, according to experimental studies [10, 12], there is a local anesthetic uptake into the CSF after diffusion through the meninges as well as an uptake into the systemic circulation after diffusion through the capillary vessel wall and a distribution into epidural and dural sleeve fat. Bioavailability in the CSF of epidurally administrated local anesthetics is low (<20%). Therefore, elimination from the epidural space is predominantly by uptake in the epidural blood flow.

3.3 Absorption and Elimination

After epidural administration, at least 95% of local anesthetics are taken up in the epidural veins and finally reach the systemic circulation [16]. Because local anesthetics are relatively lipid soluble, the diffusion through the endothelium seems not to be rate limiting and the absorption rate is mostly dependent on the local blood flow [17], which in turn may be influenced by the vasoactive properties of local anesthetics or by the sympathetic block that results from neuraxial blockade.

A biphasic absorption profile has been confirmed by many studies investigating the absorption kinetics after epidurally administered local anesthetics [18–21].

A rapid initial phase probably caused by the high initial concentration gradient is followed by a slower second phase. After systemic absorption local anesthetics are rapidly distributed to the highly perfused organs (lung, kidney, etc.) and more slowly to the less perfused tissues, such as skeletal muscle and fat [9]. The amide local anesthetics are relatively lipophilic compounds; therefore, their tissue distribution is highly dependent upon tissue perfusion.

Biotransformation and clearance of amide-type local anesthetics can be attributed almost entirely to the liver [22]. Renal excretion of an unchanged drug accounts only for less than 1–5% of the total clearance [23].

There is no or negligible metabolism of amide-type local anesthetics in the epidural and subarachnoid space, nor evidence for an extra-hepatic site of metabolism, except for prilocaine and lidocaine.

The hepatic clearance of amide-type local anesthetics is influenced in turn by liver blood flow, intrinsic enzymatic activity of liver tissue, and protein binding. Elimination of local anesthetics with a high extraction ratio such as etidocaine, lidocaine, and mepivacaine depends largely on the liver blood flow, whereas those with a low extraction ratio, such as bupivacaine and ropivacaine, depend on protein binding and enzyme activity. Clearance of an unbound drug is flow and binding dependent for high-extraction and dependent on enzyme activity for low-extraction local anesthetics [17].

Anatomical and physiological changes, associated with increasing age, may affect the pharmacokinetics of epidurally administered local anesthetics. Changes in body composition, drug binding, hepatic blood flow, and hepatic mass that occur with normal aging may have an impact on the rate and extent of the systemic absorption, distribution, metabolism, and excretion of local anesthetics.

3.4 Spread of a Solution in the Epidural Space

3.4.1 Patient Characteristics

3.4.1.1 Age
It is commonly believed that there is a positive correlation between age and spread of injected solutions into the epidural space.

This correlation could be explained by decreased leakage of local anesthetic solutions through the intervertebral foramina in older patients, even if this has been questioned [24–27].

One additional explanation is that the compliance of the epidural space increases with age, and positively correlates with the spread of the sensory block. There is a significant correlation between the epidural pressure immediately after completion of the injection, spread of analgesia, and age: the lower the epidural pressure associated with higher age, the wider the spread of analgesia [28].

Indeed the epidural space becomes more widely patent after the injection of a given amount of air during epiduroscopy, and the fatty tissue in the epidural space diminishes with increasing age, which may favor the longitudinal spread of local anesthetic solutions in the elderly [29].

Morphologic studies have reported a loss of myelinated and unmyelinated nerve fibers in elderly subjects, and several abnormalities involving myelinated fibers, such as demyelination, remyelination, and myelin balloon figures. The deterioration of myelin sheaths during aging may be due to a decrease in the expression of the major myelin proteins and may affect the functional and electrophysiological properties of the peripheral nervous system, including a decline in nerve conduction velocity, muscle strength, sensory discrimination, autonomic responses, and endoneurial blood flow [30]. These abnormalities may allow local anesthetics to more easily penetrate nerve roots in older patients. However, from the clinical point of view, when considering lumbar epidural block, conflicting results have been published and sometimes the results were statistically significant but not clinically relevant [28, 31, 32].

3.4.1.2 Height, Weight, and Body Mass Index

The effects of patient height and weight on the spread of epidural block remain unclear. Although it seems intuitive to assume that taller patients require more local anesthetic to establish a certain level of block than shorter subjects, when investigated in lumbar epidural anesthesia, only a weak correlation was found [24, 31, 33].

In lumbar epidural anesthesia, there is no correlation between weight and spread of the sensory block [31, 34]; however, the cephalad spread is positively correlated to the body mass index in the obese pregnant women [35]. Weight, BMI, and obesity are unrelated to epidural fat content [36].

3.4.1.3 Pregnancy

Pregnancy-induced changes in the epidural structures are the following: the epidural space becomes narrow, vascular network becomes dense, blood vessels become engorged, and water content in the connective tissue increases, when compared with nonpregnant women [37] (Fig. 3.3).

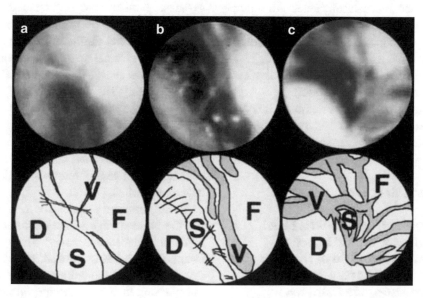

Fig. 3.3 Photographs (top) and schematic drawings (bottom) of the epidural spaces in a 32-year-old pregnant woman (**a**), in a 29-year-old woman at 12 weeks' gestation (**b**), and in a 30-year-old woman at 37 weeks' gestation (**c**). Dura mater (**d**), fatty tissue (**f**), epidural space (S), and blood vessels (V) can be observed. Engorged blood vessels appeared in the first trimester. The pneumatic space became narrow and the vascular networks became dense in the third trimester (from [37] with permission)

As pregnancy progresses, gravid uterine growth may partially obstruct the inferior vena cava in the supine position, and the epidural venous flow, collateral to the inferior vena cava, further increases. The engorged venous plexus is observed only in the anterior and lateral epidural space, and not in the posterior epidural space [37–39].

Because the engorged venous plexus in the lateral epidural space induces narrowing of the bilateral foramina at the disc level, leakage of solution injected into the epidural space from the foramen may be directly obstructed [38]. In addition, the inward pressure from the increase in the pressure in the retroperitoneal area due to pregnancy contributes to a decrease of epidural solution leakage from the foramina. Similarly, the increased inward pressure might limit dural sac coating, even in the anterior epidural space, a closed compartment that is crowded with the engorged veins, which are not rigid and easily compressive. This restricted distribution of solutions injected epidurally may explain the facilitated longitudinal spread of epidural analgesia in pregnant women [40].

However the facilitated spread of epidural analgesia occurs even during early pregnancy, at a time when mechanical factors are unlikely to play a major role [41]; therefore the hormonal changes of pregnancy should also be considered, particularly the increase in progesterone levels, that may alter the susceptibility of the nerve membrane to local anesthetics [42].

In general, for all these reasons, less local anesthetic is required to produce a given level of epidural anesthesia in pregnant patients.

3.4.2   Technical Factors

3.4.2.1 Needle Insertion Site, Bevel Orientation and Injection Through Needle or Through Catheter, Needle Bevel Direction, and Catheter Position

Differences in the pattern of epidural spread of contrast media solutions in relation to the site of injection (cervical, thoracic, or lumbar) have been noted, it being easier for the epidural solution injected into the lumbar region to spread cranially rather than caudally, but no differences were found among different regions in the total number of segments blocked [43]. The length of the lumbar section of the vertebral column is relatively short and the dimensions of the lumbar epidural space are fairly constant and only small differences in the cranial spread of the blockade have been demonstrated after the injection of local anesthetic solutions at three different lumbar interspaces [44].

The small distance between the upside and downside of the needle (usually approximately 1.2 mm in an 18-gauge Tuohy needle) may hardly influence the spread of the epidural solution when injected directly through the needle.

Whether differences may exist when the epidural solutions are injected through the catheter rather than through the needle is controversial.

Lumbar epidural bolus injection via either a Tuohy needle or a catheter did not result in differences in the epidural spread of the local anesthetic solution or the contrast medium in one study [45], whereas, in another study [46], injection through a lumbar epidural catheter resulted in a spread of sensory block four segments greater when compared to injection at the same rate through the Tuohy needle. Furthermore, a better quality of anesthesia for cesarean section was observed when the local anesthetic was injected via an epidural catheter [47].

In pregnant women, insertion of an epidural catheter with the bevel of the Tuohy needle oriented laterally may result in greater difficulty passing the catheter and, more frequently, paresthesia, but with no differences in the incidence of asymmetric block [48].

It is commonly believed that by orienting the beveled edge of the epidural needle the epidural catheter may most likely follow the intended, cephalad or caudad, direction. Indeed less than 50% of the epidural catheters that had been advanced 5 cm into the lumbar epidural space through a cephalad-directed Tuohy needle reached the intended spinal level cranial to the puncture site, most likely because many structures within the epidural space may dislodge and divert the catheters during their advancement [49].

The optimal distance to advance a (multi-orifice) catheter into the lumbar epidural space is 4–6 cm since threading shorter or longer distances may result in inadequate analgesia most likely because some segments remain unblocked due to the failure of an adequate spread of local anesthetic within the epidural space [50, 51].

Initial insertion of excessive amounts of catheter may, in addition, lead to deviations in direction, coiling, curling, kinking, or doubling back; therefore lumbar epidural catheters should not usually be threaded more than 5 cm into the epidural space [52].

Fortunately, computed tomography imaging and clinical experience demonstrate that a large variety of lumbar epidural catheter tip positions and solution distribution result in equally satisfactory epidural anesthesia [53].

3.4.2.2 Patient Position

There are no differences in maximal cranial spread if equal amounts of epidural local anesthetic solutions for labor analgesia are injected in the sitting or supine position [54].

Lumbar epidural injection of local anesthetic with the patient in the lateral position produces sensory block levels approximately 0–3 segments greater on the dependent side compared to injection with the patient in the supine position [55–61].

The head down (Trendelenburg) position of 15° may improve cephalad sensory block levels with faster onset times after lumbar epidural injection of the local anesthetic solution for cesarean section [62].

3.4.2.3 Epidural Catheter Design

In general, epidural catheters may be categorized as either single-orifice or multiorifice designs. In vitro, differential flow has been observed from multiorifice epidural catheters in as much as the flow appears first at the proximal, then the middle, and finally the distal orifices [63]. With low injection pressures, such as those generated by a continuous infusion pump, flow is largest from the proximal orifice, and no flow was observed

from the distal orifice, rendering a multiorifice catheter effectively a single-orifice variant. Comparisons between these two catheter designs are commonly presented as differences in the quality of analgesia, rather than differences in the spread of sensory block. In this regard, multiorifice catheters have been shown to be superior to single-orifice catheters in obstetric lumbar epidural anesthesia [64–66].

From the clinical point of view, it is controversial whether unilateral analgesia and unblocked segments occur more frequently when a single-orifice catheter is used, even with the newer wire-reinforced flexible catheters [66–69].

The relationship between the catheter position and the patterns of circumferential distribution of solution injected during routine epidural anesthesia has been studied through computed tomography imaging [53].

Most of the catheter tips are located in the anterior or lateral epidural space, and there is a great variability of solution distribution, which has, however, a more uniform spread with larger volume injection. The solutions injected into the complex anatomy of the epidural space travel in patterns most likely determined by the subtle pressures that force the various opposing surfaces together. In clinical practice, however, so different sites of catheter tips and spread of injected solutions are anyway compatible with adequate anesthetic effect.

Epidural catheter design may affect the peak pressure generated by epidural infusion pumps (higher with the multiorifice catheter compared to the single-orifice catheter at any delivery speeds) but whether these differences in the delivery speed of the anesthetic solution into the epidural space may correlate with differences in the duration and quality of analgesia during programmed intermittent epidural bolus delivery is still not clear [70].

3.4.2.4 Mode of Administration of the Solution

Solutions usually spread freely, although not necessarily uniformly, through the epidural space. Patterns of distribution differ greatly between patients, including uniform coating of the dural sac or preferential accumulation in the anterior or posterolateral areas, as well as variable amounts of passage out of the foramina. Injection of an additional solution after the initial single bolus improves the uniformity of distribution [53]. After a single epidural bolus the injectate solution disperses widely throughout the epidural space in both caudal and rostral directions, with a predominantly rostral spread [71]. When the bolus has been injected at a flow rate that mimics that used for the injection of local anesthetics in clinical practice, there is a rapid spread of the epidural solution from the epidural space into the paravertebral tissues. This relatively high-flow-rate bolus may produce sufficiently high local pressures to permit the leakage of fluid along nerve roots passing through the spinal foramina into the paravertebral tissues [53]. Administration of a fixed-volume, single manual bolus produces a greater longitudinal extent of circumferential spread, compared to the delivery of the same volume via a mechanical infusion [72]. Bolus injection rates via mechanical pumps are generally slower and injection pressures generally lower than manual boluses; however the same results, in terms

of diffusion of the epidural solutions, have been obtained using pumps instead of manual administration in order to better control the bolus flow rate.

When an intermittent bolus technique is used, the spread of the infuscate from a multiorifice catheter is better, resulting in a wider and more uniform spread of contrast medium, while the continuous infusion results in a smaller spread that is exclusively through the proximal port of the epidural catheter [73–76]. Studies of cadaveric and pregnant women support the theory that a more uniform spread of the solution in the epidural space could be achieved as a result of the higher injectate pressure generated during a bolus injection. Indeed, in cadaveric studies, the spread of fluids in the epidural space is highly nonuniform in multiple small channels and it is more uniform in large volumes given in high injectate pressure near the site of injection which will result in engagement of most of the channels [75] (Figs. 3.4 and 3.5).

When an automated intermittent bolus is associated with combined epidural spinal anesthesia (CSE) the intrathecal space could directly receive

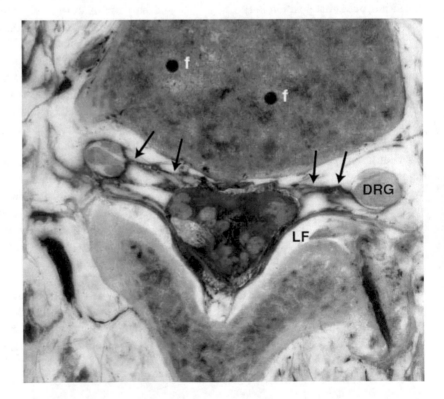

Fig. 3.4 Axial cryomicrotome image at the level of the fourth lumbar vertebra and spinal nerve. Green ink passes through the intervertebral foramina as multiple channels between lobules of fat, limited by the ligamentum flavum (LF) and fascia or the posterior longitudinal ligament (black arrows), which guides solution to the segmental nerve and dorsal root ganglion (DRG) (from [75] with permission)

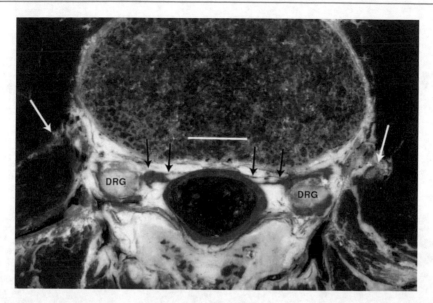

Fig. 3.5 Axial cryomicrotome image at the level of the third and fourth lumbar vertebra. Orange ink is seen as an accumulation circumferentially around the dura, with laminar extensions into the intervertebral foramina along the posterior aspect of the fascia of the posterior longitudinal ligament (black arrows). The injectate also tracks with the segmental nerve, shown here at the level of the dorsal root ganglia (DRG). More cephalad components of the lumbar plexus are evident in the substance of the psoas muscle (white arrows) (from [75] with permission)

the local anesthetic solution through the dural rent, owing to the high driving pressure created when the bolus is administered, so leading to a more efficacious analgesia [77].

In vitro, the pressure generated by an infusion pump is consistently higher when it is set to give the same volume of an epidural solution as a bolus rather than as a continuous infusion, and this may suggest that the mode of delivery of a solution plays an important role in determining its distribution in the epidural space [78]. This has been confirmed by the in vivo measurements of the epidural pressures in pregnant patients, which clearly demonstrate the greater pressures generated in the epidural space by an automated bolus technique when compared to a continuous infusion [76].

In general, higher programmed intermittent epidural bolus infusion delivery speeds result in higher peak pressure generation; however whether differences in the infusion delivery speed correlate with differences in the epidural spread is not clear [70].

The way of delivering analgesia by single bolus or by continuous infusion may subse-quently influence the dynamics of nerve block. As stated in pharmacodynamics, the movement of local anesthetic into the nerve according to diffusion gradients can determine the production and reversal of analgesia and motor block [79].

Analgesia and motor block are produced by the movement of local anesthetic from the extraneural space into the nerve along a diffusion gradient. After a single bolus administration, the concentration is initially greater outside of the nerve fiber but over time the extraneural concentration equals the intraneural one, establishing a steady state. Nerve blockade is eventually overcome when the intraneural concentration exceeds the extraneural concentration and the diffusion gradient is reversed. If a local anesthetic at very low concentration is used in intermittent boluses, the amount of local anesthetic inside the nerve fiber is sufficient to block the sensory fibers, which are small and with a short internodal distance, but the blockade of motor fibers, which are greater and with a long internodal distance, is unlikely, as the total amount of local anesthetic inside the nerve is insufficient to block them. In the case of continuous infusion, the extraneural concentration

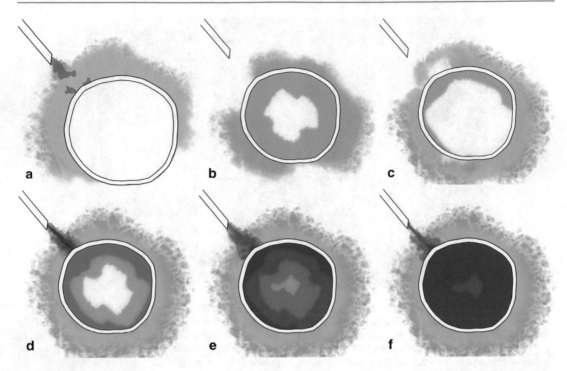

Fig. 3.6 Dynamics after a single bolus administration. (**a**) Initially the concentration is greater outside of the nerve fiber. (**b**) Over time the extraneural concentration equals the intraneural one, establishing a steady state. (**c**) Nerve blockade is eventually overcome when the intraneural concentration exceeds the extraneural concentra-tion and the diffusion gradient is reversed. Dynamics after continuous infusion. (**d**) The extraneural concentration of local anesthetic is generally constantly higher than in the intraneural space. (**e**, **f**) The total concentration inside the nerve is increased with time and may reach the threshold for motor fiber block

of local anesthetic is generally constantly higher than in the intraneural space, and the total concentration inside the nerve is therefore increased over time and may reach the threshold for motor fiber block even if we are using a local anesthetic solution at very low concentration (Fig. 3.6).

This may explain the frequent occurrence and intensification of motor block during prolonged continuous infusions like those used for labor analgesia.

3.4.2.5 Speed of Injection

The spread of injection correlates with the peak epidural pressure generated by the injection, being higher with faster injections, but does not correlate with the extent and regression of the sensory block [80]. This is also observed in animal studies where the peak of the epidural

pressure is directly correlated with the injection speed of the epidural solution but not with the epidural distribution and extent of sensory block [81].

In vitro studies also confirm this finding. Using a pump designed for programmed intermittent infusion boluses, the delivery speed of saline solution through epidural catheters is directly related to the peak pressures. However it is not known whether differences in the delivery speed of anesthetic solution into the epidural space correlate with differences in the duration and quality of analgesia during programmed intermittent epidural bolus delivery [70].

It seems that the only feature that can be obtained by a fast speed of injection of the epidural solution is the earlier establishment of the block [46, 82].

3.4.3 Epidural Pressure and Adjacent Pressures

There was a debate in the earlier studies as to whether epidural pressure was positive or negative (with regard to atmosphere) or if it was an artifact caused by devices used to explore the space [83–85].

It is now clear that there is no naturally occurring negative pressure in the lumbar epidural space and that the negative pressure, sometimes recorded, is an artifact resulting from bulging of the ligamentum flavum in advance of the needle with its rapid return to the resting position once perforated [86].

In pregnancy, during labor and during the postpartum period the epidural space pressure is above atmospheric and its actual values may vary from 4 up to 30 mmHg, depending on the measurement techniques used and other variables, such as patient position and whether she is in labor or not [76, 87, 88].

The epidural pressure is higher in the supine position than in the lateral position with the patient horizontal. This difference may be due to the fact that in the supine position the right atrium lies on average 8 cm higher than the internal vertebral plexus, but the most important factor is the degree of inferior vena cava occlusion. During labor there is a significant rise in epidural pressure synchronous with the intrauterine pressure wave of contractions and this increase is even most significant in the supine position or in the case of twin pregnancy.

However this increase of pressure synchronous with the uterine contractions is dependent upon the parturient's awareness of contraction and upon her muscular response to it. When the parturient is in pain she contracts her abdominal muscles, causing an increase in intra-abdominal pressure, which in turn results in a further impediment to the flow in the inferior vena cava and a consequent rise in the epidural pressure. When the mother is under epidural analgesia and unaware of the uterine contractions, this sequence of events does not occur, and the synchronous increase in epidural pressure is of a lower extent. If in addition to abolition of awareness of contraction (anesthesia) there is also an abdominal muscle paralysis (extensive motor block), there is a fall in the epidural pressure synchronous with uterine contraction when the parturient is in the lateral position. This drop of pressure is most likely due to the absence of resistance offered by the paralyzed abdominal muscles to the contracting uterus, permitting the latter to fall away from the spine, thereby improving the blood flow in the inferior vena cava. Also the "tenting" of the abdominal wall by the contracting uterus will cause the intra-abdominal pressure to drop and engorgement of the epidural veins will be reduced. The resulting increase in the epidural space capacity will cause its pressure to drop.

During the contractions the epidural pressure remains approximately sustained throughout labor. During the second stage of labor with the patient bearing down in the semi-sitting position the epidural pressure increases. At the end of the third stage, the obstruction of the inferior vena cava is alleviated; venous blood that was diverted to the epidural veins before and during labor is redirected back into its normal path; and the capacity of epidural space increases and its pressure decreases. The magnitude of this drop is related to the length of labor and the mode of delivery.

Pressure gradients within the epidural space, and between this space and adjacent body cavities, may also play a role in the distribution of local anesthetic solutions injected in the epidural space.

The increase in pressure in the retroperitoneal area due to pregnancy generates an inward pressure on the fat around the intervertebral foramina, limiting the epidural solution leakage from the foramina themselves. This restricted distribution of solutions injected epidurally may contribute to explain the facilitated longitudinal spread of epidural analgesia in pregnant women [40].

3.4.4 Composition of the Solution Injected: Dose, Volume, and Concentration—Adjuvant Drugs

Generally speaking, the primary qualities of epidural anesthesia such as onset, depth, and duration of the block are related to the mass of drug administered.

As the dose of the local anesthetic increases, the frequency of satisfactory anesthesia and the duration of anesthesia increase and the time for onset of anesthesia decreases. In general, the dose of local anesthetic given may be increased by administering a larger volume of a less concentrated solution or a smaller volume of a more concentrated solution. In clinical practice, however, an increase in dosage is usually achieved by using a more concentrated solution of a specific local anesthetic agent.

Administration of the same mass of local anesthetics in larger volumes results in a greater spread of the solution [89, 90]; however, the intensity of block decreases as the volume of the solution increases (and the concentration of local anesthetic decreases).

Although the volume of the anesthetic solution administered into the epidural space may influence the cephalic spread of anesthesia, the relationship between spread and volume of the anesthetic solution is neither lineal nor predictable [1].

An increase in pH by adding bicarbonate to a solution of local anesthetic results in an increase in the nonionized fraction of the local anesthetic and improves the nerve penetration.

Alkalization of the solution may increase the pain threshold in blocked dermatomes, and the depth of motor block, and reduce the time to onset of blockade of the first sacral segment, but does not affect the spread of the block [91].

Adding opioids to epidural local anesthetic may also hasten the onset, but does not affect the spread of the anesthetic solution and therefore the spread of sensory block [92].

References

1. Bromage PR. Spread of analgesic solutions in the epidural space and their site of action: a statistical study. Br J Anaesth. 1962;34:161–78.
2. Bromage PR. Mechanisms of action. In: Bromage PR, editor. Epidural analgesia. Philadelphia: W.B. Saunders; 1978.
3. Hogan Q, Toth J. Anatomy of soft tissues of the spinal canal. Reg Anesth Pain Med. 1999;24:303–10.
4. Bernards CM, Hill HF. The spinal nerve root sleeve is not a preferred route for redistribution of drugs from the epidural space to spinal cord. Anesthesiology. 1991;75:827–32.
5. Covino BG. Pharmacology of local anaesthetic agents. Br J Anaesth. 1986;58:701–16.
6. Tucker GT, Mather LE. Pharmacology of local anaesthetic agents. Pharmacokinetics of local anaesthetic agents. Br J Anaesth Suppl. 1975;47:213–24.
7. Strichartz GR, Sanchez V, Arthur GR, et al. Fundamental properties of local anaesthetics. II. Measured octanol: buffer partition coefficients and pKa values of clinically used drugs. Anesth Analg. 1990;71:158–70.
8. Tucker GT, Mather LE. Properties, absorption, and disposition of local anesthetic agents. In: Cousins MJ, Bridenbaugh PO, editors. Neural blockade in clinical anesthesia and management of pain. 3rd ed. Philadelphia: Lippincott-Raven Publishers; 1998. p. 55–95.
9. Veering BT. Clinical pharmacology of local anaesthetics. In: Rosenberg P, editor. Fundamentals of anaesthesia and acute medicine: local and regional anaesthesia. London: BMJ Publishing Group; 2000. p. 1–2.
10. Clement R, Malinovsky JM, Hildgen P, et al. Spinal disposition and meningeal permeability of local anaesthetics. Pharm Res. 2004;21:706–16.
11. Bernards CM, Hill HF. Physical and chemical properties of drug molecules governing their diffusion through the spinal meninges. Anesthesiology. 1992;77:750–6.
12. Clement R, Malinovsky JM, Le Corre P, et al. Cerebrospinal fluid bioavailability and pharmacokinetics of bupivacaine and lidocaine after intrathecal and epidural administrations in rabbits using micro dialysis. J Pharmacol Exp Ther. 1999;289:1015–21.
13. Bernards CM. Sophistry in medicine: lessons from the epidural space. Reg Anesth Pain Med. 2005;30:56–66.
14. Reina MA, Franco CD, López A, et al. Clinical implications of epidural fat in the spinal canal. A scanning electron microscopic study. Acta Anaesth Belg. 2009;60:7–17.
15. Zenker W, Bankoul S, Braun JS. Morphological indications for considerable diffuse reabsorption of cerebrospinal fluid in spinal meninges particularly in the areas of meningeal funnels. An electron microscopical study including tracing experiments in rats. Anat Embryol. 1994;189:243–58.
16. Burm AGL. Clinical pharmacokinetics of epidural and spinal anaesthesia. Clin Pharmacokinet. 1989;16:283–311.
17. Tucker GT. Pharmacokinetics of local anaesthetics. Br J Anaesth. 1986;58:717–31.
18. Burm AGL, Vermeulen NP, van Kleef JW, et al. Pharmacokinetics of lignocaine and bupivacaine in surgical patients following epidural administration. Simultaneous investigation of absorption

and disposition kinetics using stable isotopes. Clin Pharmacokinet. 1987;13:191–203.

19. Veering BT, Burm AGL, Vletter AA, et al. The effect of age on the systemic absorption, disposition and pharmacodynamics of bupivacaine after epidural administration. Clin Pharmacokinet. 1992;22:75–84.

20. Simon MJG, Veering BT, Stienstra R, et al. The systemic absorption and disposition of levobupivacaine 0.5% after epidural administration in surgical patients: a stable-isotope study. Eur J Anaesthesiol. 2004;21:460–70.

21. Simon MJG, Veering BT, Stienstra R, et al. Effect of age on the clinical profile and systemic absorption and disposition of levobupivacaine after epidural administration. Br J Anaesth. 2004;93:512–20.

22. Veering BT, Burm AGL. Pharmacokinetics and pharmacodynamics of medullar agents. 3a. Local anaesthetics. Baillieres Clin Anaesthesiol. 1993;7:557–77.

23. Tucker GT, Mather LE. Clinical pharmacokinetics of local anaesthetics. Clin Pharmacokinet. 1979;4:241–78.

24. Park WY, Massengale MD, Kim SI, et al. Age and the spread of local anesthetic solutions in the epidural space. Anesth Analg. 1980;59:768–71.

25. Ferrer-Brechner T. Spinal and epidural anesthesia in the elderly. Semin Anesth. 1986;5:54–61.

26. Shanta TR, Evans JA. The relationship of epidural anesthesia to neural membranes and arachnoid villi. Anesthesiology. 1972;37:543–57.

27. Saitoh K, Hirabayashi Y, Shimizu R, et al. Extensive extradural spread in the elderly may not relate to decreased leakage through intervertebral foramina. Br J Anaesth. 1995;75:688–91.

28. Hirabayashi Y, Matsuda I, Sohzaburoh I, et al. Spread of epidural analgesia following a constant pressure injection-an investigation of relationships between locus of injection, epidural pressure and spread of analgesia. J Anesth. 1987;1:44–50.

29. Igarashi T, Hirabayashi Y, Shimizu R, et al. The lumbar extradural structure changes with increasing age. Br J Anaesth. 1997;78:149–52.

30. Verdu E, Ceballos D, Vilches JJ, et al. Influence of aging on peripheral nerve function and regeneration. J Peripher Nerv Syst. 2000;5:191–208.

31. Duggan J, Bowler GM, McClure JH, et al. Extradural block with bupivacaine: influence of dose, volume, concentration and patient characteristics. Br J Anaesth. 1988;61:324–31.

32. Andersen S, Cold GE. Dose response studies in elderly patients subjected to epidural analgesia. Acta Anaesthesiol Scand. 1981;25:279–81.

33. Grundy EM, Ramamurthy S, Patel KP, et al. Extradural analgesia revisited: a statistical study. Br J Anaesth. 1978;50:805–9.

34. Whalley DG, D'Amico JA, Rybicki LA, et al. The effect of posture on the induction of epidural anesthesia for peripheral vascular surgery. Reg Anesth. 1995;20:407–11.

35. Hodkinson R, Husain FJ. Obesity and the cephalad spread of analgesia following epidural administration of bupivacaine for cesarean section. Anesth Analg. 1980;59:89–92.

36. Alicioglu B, Sarac A, Tokuc B. Does abdominal obesity cause increase in the amount of epidural fat? Eur Spine J. 2008;17:1324–8.

37. Igarashi T, Hirabayashi Y, Shimizu R, et al. The fiberscopic findings of the epidural space in pregnant women. Anesthesiology. 2000;92:1631–6.

38. Takiguchi T, Yamaguchi S, Tezuka M, et al. Compression of the subarachnoid space by the engorged epidural venous plexus in pregnant women. Anesthesiology. 2006;105:848–51.

39. Onuki E, Higuchi H, Takagi S, et al. Gestation-related reduction in lumbar cerebrospinal fluid volume and dural sac surface area. Anesth Analg. 2010;110:148–53.

40. Higuchi H, Takagi S, Onuki E, et al. Distribution of epidural saline upon injection and the epidural volume effect in pregnant women. Anesthesiology. 2011;114:1155–61.

41. Fagraeus L, Urban BJ, Bromage PR. Spread of epidural analgesia in early pregnancy. Anesthesiology. 1983;58:184–7.

42. Datta S, Hurley RJ, Naulty IS, et al. Plasma and cerebrospinal fluid progesterone concentrations in pregnant and nonpregnant women. Anesth Analg. 1986;65:950–4.

43. Visser WA, Liem TH, van Egmond J, et al. Extension of sensory blockade after thoracic administration of a test dose of lidocaine at three different levels. Anesth Analg. 1998;86:332–5.

44. Curatolo M, Orlando A, Zbinden AM, et al. A multifactorial analysis of the spread of epidural analgesia. Acta Anesthesiol Scand. 1994;38:646–52.

45. Yun MJ, Kim YC, Lim YJ, et al. The differential flow of epidural local anaesthetic via needle or catheter: a prospective randomized double-blind study. Anaesth Intensive Care. 2004;32:377–82.

46. Omote K, Namiki A, Iwasaki H. Epidural administration and analgesic spread: comparison of injection with catheters and needles. J Anesth. 1992;6:289–93.

47. Crochetiere CT, Trepanier CA, Cote JJ. Epidural anaesthesia for caesarean section: comparison of two injection techniques. Can J Anaesth. 1989;36:133–6.

48. Richardson MG, Wissler RN. The effects of needle bevel orientation during epidural catheter insertion in laboring parturients. Anesth Analg. 1999;88:352–6.

49. Beck H. The effect of the Tuohy cannula on the positioning of an epidural catheter. A radiologic analysis of the location of 175 peridural catheters. Reg Anaesth. 1990;13:42–5.

50. Beilin Y, Bernstein HH, Zucker-Pinchoff B. The optimal distance that a multiorifice epidural catheter should be threaded into the epidural space. Anesth Analg. 1995;81:301–4.

51. D'Angelo R, Berkebile B, Gerancher JC. Prospective examination of epidural catheter insertion. Anesthesiology. 1996;84:88–93.

52. Muneyuki M, Shirai K, Inamoto A. Roentgenographic analysis of the positions of catheters in the epidural space. Anesthesiology. 1970;33:19–24.

53. Hogan Q. Epidural catheter tip position and distribution of injectate evaluated by computed tomography. Anesthesiology. 1999;90:964–70.

54. Redick LF. The effect of patient position and obesity on the spread of epidural analgesia. Int J Obstet Anesth. 1993;3:134–6.

55. Grundy EM, Rao LN, Winnie AP. Epidural anesthesia and the lateral position. Anesth Analg. 1978;57:95–7.

56. Apostolou GA, Zarmakoupis PK, Mastrokostopoulos GT. Spread of epidural anesthesia and the lateral position. Anesth Analg. 1981;60:584–6.

57. Husemeyer RP, White DC. Lumbar extradural injection pressures in pregnant women: an investigation of relationships between rate of injection, injection pressures, and extent of analgesia. Br J Anaesth. 1980;52:55–60.

58. Park WY, Hagins FM, Macnamara TE. Lateral position and epidural anesthetic spread. Anesth Analg. 1983;62:278–9.

59. Preston R, Crosby ET, Kotarba D, et al. Maternal positioning affects fetal heart rate changes after epidural analgesia for labour. Can J Anaesth. 1993;40:1136–41.

60. Soetens FM, Meeuwis HC, van der Donck AG, et al. Influence of maternal position during epidural labor analgesia. Int J Obstet Anesth. 2003;12:98–101.

61. Shapiro A, Fredman B, Zohar E, et al. Alternating patient position following the induction of obstetric epidural analgesia does not affect local anaesthetic spread. Int J Obstet Anesth. 1998;7:153–6.

62. Setayesh AR, Kholdebarin AR, Saber Moghadam M, et al. The Trendelenburg position increases the spread and accelerates the onset of epidural anesthesia for cesarean section. Can J Anaesth. 2001;48:890–3.

63. Power I, Thorburn J. Differential flow from multihole epidural catheters. Anaesthesia. 1988;43:876–8.

64. Segal S, Eappen S, Datta S. Superiority of multiorifice over single-orifice epidural catheters for labor analgesia and cesarean section. J Clin Anesth. 1997;9:109–12.

65. D'Angelo R, Foss ML, Livesay CH. A comparison of multiport and uniport epidural catheters in laboring patients. Anesth Analg. 1997;84:1276–9.

66. Michael S, Richmond MN, Livesay CH. A comparison between open end (single hole) and closed end (three lateral holes) epidural catheters. Anaesthesia. 1988;44:78–80.

67. Morrison LM, Buchan AS. Comparison of complications associated with single-holed and multi-holed extradural catheters. Br J Anaesth. 1990;64:183–5.

68. Magides AD, Sprigg A, Richmond MN. Lumbar epidurography with multi-orifice and single-orifice catheters. Anaesthesia. 1996;51:757–63.

69. Philip J, Sharma SK, Sparks TJ, et al. Multiple ports do not appear to improve the analgesic efficacy of wire-reinforced flexible catheters used for LEA. Anesth Analg. 2018;126:537–44.

70. Klumpner TT, Lange EM, Ahmed HS, et al. An in vitro evaluation of the pressure generated during programmed intermittent epidural bolus injection at varying infusion delivery speeds. J Clin Anesth. 2016;34:632–7.

71. Paisley K, Jeffries J, Monroe M, et al. Dispersal pattern of injectate after lumbar interlaminar epidural spinal injection. Evaluation with computerized tomography. Global Spine J. 2012;2:27–32.

72. Mowatt I, Tang R, Vaghadia H at al. Epidural distribution of dye administered via an epidural catheter in a porcine model. Br J Anaesth. 2016;116:277–81.

73. Fettes PDW, Moore CS, Whiteside JB, et al. Intermittent vs continuous administration of epidural ropivacaine with fentanyl for analgesia during labour. Br J Anaesth. 2006;97:359–64.

74. Kaynar AM, Shankar KB. Epidural infusion: continuous or bolus? Anesth Analg. 1999;89:534.

75. Hogan Q. Distribution of solution in the epidural space: examination by cryomicrotome section. Reg Anesth Pain Med. 2002;27:150–66.

76. Gibiino G, Distefano R, Camorcia M, et al. Maternal epidural pressure changes after programmed intermittent epidural bolus (PIEB) versus continuous epidural infusion (CEI). Eur J Anaesth. 2014;31:11AP35.

77. Chua SM, Sia AT. Automated intermittent epidural boluses improve analgesia induced by intrathecal fentanyl during labour. Can J Anaesth. 2004;51:581–5.

78. Stirparo S, Fortini S, Espa S, et al. An in vitro evaluation of pressure generated by programmed intermittent epidural bolus (PIEB) or continuous epidural infusion (CEI). Open J Anesthesiol. 2013;3:214 7.

79. De Jong RH. Dynamics of nerve block. In: De Jong RH, editor. Local anesthetics. St Louis: Mosby; 1994. p. 230–45.

80. Cardoso M, Carvalho JCA. Epidural pressures and spread of 2% lidocaine in the epidural space: influence of volume and spread of injection of the local anesthetic solution. RAPM. 1998;23:14–9.

81. Son W, Jang M, Yoon J, et al. The effect of epidural injection speed on epidural pressure and distribution of solution in anesthetized dogs. Vet Anesth Analg. 2016;41:526–33.

82. Griffiths RB, Horton WA, Jones IG, et al. Spread of injection and spread of bupivacaine in the epidural space. Anaesthesia. 1987;42:160–3.

83. Heldt HJ, Moloney JC. Negative pressure in the epidural space. Am J Med Sci. 1928;175:371–6.

84. Usubiaga JE, Moya F, Usubiaga LE. Effect of thoracic and abdominal pressure changes on the epidural space pressure. Br J Anaesth. 1967;39:612–8.

85. Bromage PR. Epidural pressure. In: Bromage PR, editor. Epidural analgesia. Saunders Co: Philadelphia; 1978. p. 160–75.

86. Zarzur E. Genesis of the 'true' negative pressure in the lumbar epidural space. Anaesthesia. 1984;39:1101–4.

87. Galbert MW, Marx GF. Extradural pressures in the parturient patient. Anesthesiology. 1974;40:499–502.
88. Messih MNA. Epidural space pressures during pregnancy. Anaesthesia. 1981;36:775–82.
89. Okutomi T, Minakawa M, Hoka S. Saline volume and local anesthetic concentration modify the spread of epidural anesthesia. Can J Anaesth. 1999;46:930–4.
90. Burn JM, Guyer PB, Langdon L. The spread of solutions injected into the epidural space. Br J Anaesth. 1973;54:338–45.
91. Arakawa M, Aoyama Y, Ohe Y. Epidural bolus injection with alkalinized lidocaine improves blockade of the first sacral segment—a brief report. Can J Anaesth. 2002;49:566–70.
92. Cherng CH, Yang CP, Wong CS. Epidural fentanyl speeds the onset of sensory and motor blocks during epidural ropivacaine anesthesia. Anesth Analg. 2005;101:1834–7.

Early pioneers used spinal needles to perform the epidural block. Achille Dogliotti (1897–1966), professor of surgery in Turin, for example, suggested the use of a 0.8–1 mm diameter needle, slightly larger than those used for the subarachnoid puncture, with a short, blunt tip to reduce the danger of puncturing the dura mater [1] (Fig. 1.6).

In 1931, in order to prolong the single-shot epidural procedure, Eugen Aburel (1899–1975) [2], professor of obstetrics in Romania, introduced a continuous lumboaortic block with a silk ureteral catheter for labor analgesia.

In the 1940s, William Lemmon (1896–1974) [3] developed a malleable needle to provide continuous spinal anesthesia by inserting a small rubber tube in it.

In the same period of time, a Seattle dentist, Ralph Huber (1890–1953) [4], designed a long, sharp, curved-tip hypodermic needle to lessen the pain of the injection and decrease the risk of depositing plugs of skin into underlying tissues.

Edward Tuohy (1908–1959) [5], anesthesiologist at the Mayo Clinic, recognized that the Huber needle's directional point might facilitate the placement of spinal catheters and, in addition, he added a stylet to further decrease the risk of skin plugging. Tuohy described it as a needle with a Huber point. Since then, any epidural needle with a Huber tip became known as a "Tuohy needle." After visiting the Mayo Clinic, Manuel Curbelo (1906–1962) [6], a Cuban anesthesiologist, adapted the Tuohy spinal continuous technique for the epidural space using ureteral catheters, and his technique was popularized to the obstetric population by Charles Flowers (1920–1999) [7] in Baltimore.

Approximately 10 years later, Robert Hustead (1928–2008) [8] made his own modifications to the Tuohy–Huber needle by hand, changing the angle of the bevel. The result was a needle opening that did not exceed 2.7 mm in length, with an angle of the needle bevel of 12°–15°.

In the 1950s Oral Crawford (1921–2008) in Springfield, USA, developed a Quincke-type epidural needle with an extremely short, blunt, flat bevel that he used for cervical and thoracic epidural blocks using the "hanging-drop" method to identify the epidural space [9].

The addition of "wings" to the epidural needle is attributed to Jess Weiss (1917–2007), who felt that the addition of wings was essential to allow the slow advance of the needle with both hands while observing the fluid drop disappearing as the tip of the needle entered the epidural space.

By the second half of the twentieth century the practice of epidural analgesia gained popularity worldwide and a number of innovations in design and manufacture of epidural needles, catheters, and syringes were made.

The needles currently on the market under the name of "Tuohy needle" can, however, have significantly different physical characteristics: even with the same size, the needle length, width, angulation, and bevel length may vary between manufacturers.

© Springer Nature Switzerland AG 2020
G. Capogna, *Epidural Technique In Obstetric Anesthesia*,
https://doi.org/10.1007/978-3-030-45332-9_4

The silk- or elastic gum-made ureteral catheters adapted in the past for continuous spinal and epidural techniques have now been substituted with catheters made from different materials such as nylon, polyethylene, and Teflon which have dramatically improved flexibility and textile strength.

Also syringes have undergone noticeable changes over time. From the reusable, all-glass syringes commonly employed in the 1940s, polypropylene-made, single-use, low-friction syringes are now currently available on the market, specifically designed to facilitate the successful location of the epidural space.

Differences between manufacturers of these pieces of equipment may require readjustment in tactile perception, force, and angulation entry in the epidural space by physicians.

4.1 Epidural Equipment

4.1.1 Epidural Needles

Epidural needles commonly used for the obstetric patients, and therefore for the lumbar epidural block, are very often referred to as Tuohy needles, even though variations in their tip configuration make them sometimes much closer to a Hustead needle design. In addition, bevel variations may be noted between manufacturers (Fig. 4.1).

In all cases the bevel on the needle is usually blunted to maximize the tactile feeling of the operator and slightly curved superiorly (Huber point), to direct the catheter cephalad. The length

of the bevel may range from 2.32 to 3.26 mm and the width from 1.20 to 1.34 mm. The needle angulation may range approximately between 12° and 16° and the minimum length of the bevel required for the catheter to exit the bevel may also vary from 1.0 to 1.63 mm [10].

Short-blunted, flat-beveled, Crawford-type needles, specifically designed for thoracic epidural block and for hanging-drop technique, are rarely used in obstetrics (Fig. 4.2).

The length of epidural needles available on the market may vary between 8 and 15 cm from the hub to the tip. The barrel of the needle is usually

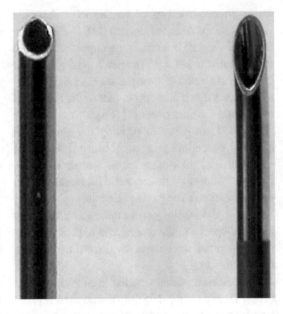

Fig. 4.2 Crawford (on the left) and Tuohy (on the right) needle

Fig. 4.1 Tuohy needles: bevel variations may be noted between manufacturers

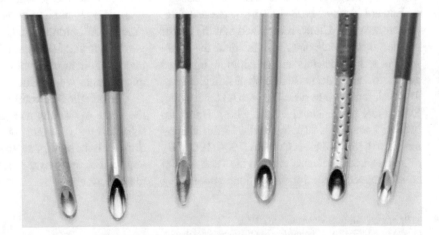

marked in graduations of 1 cm with alternating light and dark bands, so that the length of the needle already inserted may be deduced.

The thickness of the most frequently used epidural needles ranges between 16 and 19 gauge (G). The higher the gauge, the thinner the needle.

Gauges were old measures of thickness originated during the nineteenth century in the British iron wire industry at a time when there was no universal unit of thickness. At that time the gauge was a range of sizes specific to one manufacturer or branch of industry. Now it is described in fractions of an inch, but the sequence of the sizes is not linear [11]. Manufacturer differences may be noted in the inner and outer diameter of the needle, being different even within the same gauge range [12].

Some manufacturers include separate wings in their packs, and these may be connected to the needle in case the hanging-drop technique for a thoracic epidural is required [13, 14].

Others, however, provide pre-attached wings, some of which cannot be removed.

The needle has an obturator or stylet (made of stainless steel or polypropylene) which offset

tip sits flush with the tip of the needle to prevent cores of dermal tissue from being introduced into underlying tissues.

Hubs and/or stylet hubs are usually color coded, for easy identification of the size of the needle.

Significant variations between different manufacturers in needle stiffness and malleability, as assessed by buckling force and displacement, may be observed [12].

4.1.2   Epidural Syringes

Specifically designed syringes to facilitate the loss of resistance technique (LORT) are now commonly used, and many products are currently available (Fig. 4.3).

Syringes have three major uses: aspiration, identification of epidural space with LORT, and injection of the solution.

The plunger should be inserted fully into the barrel and the needle's female Luer is securely attached to the male Luer on the syringe barrel. Fluid is then

Fig. 4.3 Epidural loss of resistance (LOR) syringes

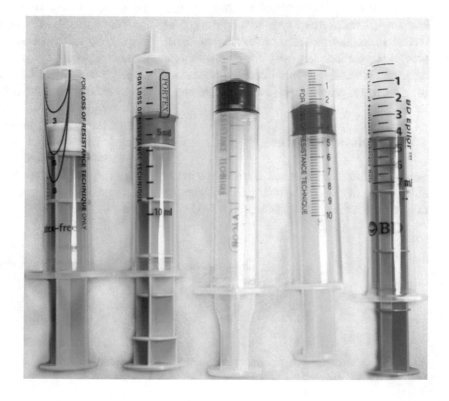

drawn up through the needle into the barrel when the plunger handle is pulled back. If the needle tip remains completely in the fluid when pulling back on the plunger handle, no air should enter the barrel. The quantity of fluid can be identified using graduation marks on the barrel, or if no marks are present, the total volume of the barrel matches the size of the LOR syringe originally identified. Pushing back on the plunger handle, the solution will be evacuated.

The standardized system of fittings which make a leak-free connection between syringe and needle is called Luer connection, after Hermann Wülfing Luer, a nineteenth-century medical instrument maker. There are two types of Luer taper connections: Luer Lock and Luer Slip. The Luer Lock holds the female Luer needle to the syringe's male Luer using threads to lock the needle to the syringe. The Luer Slip is held together by friction between the female hub taper and the male Luer taper on the syringe barrel only.

Syringes may be made of glass or of a plastic material such as polypropylene.

A modern glass loss-of-resistance syringe features a smoothly moving plunger designed to facilitate the location of the epidural space.

The plastic, single-use, loss-of-resistance syringe is a low-friction syringe specifically designed to facilitate successful location of the epidural space providing excellent sensitivity for epidural space detection. It usually features a double-ribbed stopper designed to prevent leakage during aspiration.

4.1.3 Epidural Devices

Some automated mechanical devices are available on the market in the attempt to reduce the failure rate of the epidural technique [15–17].

Unfortunately their use is reported only in a few papers, and the extent of their routine use in worldwide clinical obstetric practice is unknown, although a survey from the UK reported their use in approximately 1% of cases [18].

The automatic detection of the epidural space may be obtained by the continuous positive pressure applied to the loss of resistance syringe piston by an elastic strip (Oxford Detector, Epimatic®) (Fig. 4.4) or by an internal compression spring that applies constant pressure on the plunger (Episure™ AutoDetect™ syringe, Epi-Jet®) which automatically depresses when the needle enters the epidural space (Fig. 4.5).

When the Tuohy needle enters the epidural space, the loss of resistance is therefore made visible by the sudden inward movement of the syringe piston. The manufacturers report that with these syringes the physician can have a hand free which can be used to better control the insertion of the Tuohy needle or hold an ultrasound probe.

Epidural balloons are also available: they consist of an inflatable balloon with a capacity of 5 mL which is plugged into one end of the device, and a free end which attaches to the Tuohy needle. The balloon may be inflated through its thick rubber neck (Macintosh), or through a one-way valve (Epidural Balloon-Vygon®) (Fig. 4.6). After having advanced the Tuohy needle from the skin to the supraspinous ligament, the epidural balloon is attached to the hub of the epidural needle and the balloon is inflated with 2 mL of air. The epidural needle is eventually advanced deeper and, as the needle passes through the ligamentum flavum and enters the epidural space, the balloon becomes deflated.

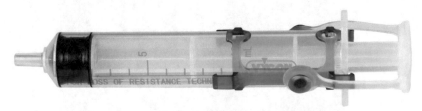

Fig. 4.4 The Epimatic® syringe: the automatic detection of the epidural space is obtained by the continuous positive pressure applied to the loss of resistance syringe piston by an elastic strip

Fig. 4.5 The Episure™
AutoDetect™ syringe
and the Epi-Jet®
syringes: an internal
compression spring
applies constant pressure
on the plunger which
automatically depresses
when the needle enters
the epidural space

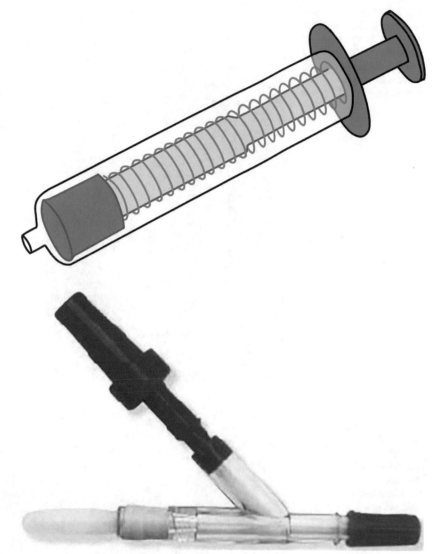

Fig. 4.6 Epidural
Balloon-Vygon®: as the
needle passes through
the ligamentum flavum
and enters the epidural
space, the balloon
becomes deflated

A modified balloon system is the Epidrum®
(Fig. 4.7), which is a device consisting of a cylindrical tube with sealed ends, which creates a chamber [19]. The seal on the top end of the tube is an
expandable membrane (the diaphragm), which
deflates when the epidural needle enters the epidural space. There are two ports, placed opposite
each other in the walls of the cylinder. The inlet
port (a female Luer), containing a nonreturn valve,
connects with a syringe and the outlet port (a male
Luer) connects with an epidural needle. After
inserting the epidural needle through the skin and
into tissue, air is drawn into a pre-connected 5 mL

Luer syringe, and 1 mL of air is injected into the
cylinder, thereby inflating the diaphragm. The
nonreturn valve ensures that air remains inside the
device. When the epidural needle tip enters the
epidural space the diaphragm deflates, signaling
to the user that the needle is in the epidural space.
The clinician will decide on the amount of air to
be injected into the chamber, which can be topped
up to a maximum of 3 mL, depending on the size
and weight of the person having the epidural, and
whether any air leakage into the tissues occurs.

Another modified balloon system is the LOR
Indicator Syringe™ [20] (Fig. 4.8). In this case

Fig. 4.7 Epidrum®: when the epidural needle tip enters the epidural space the diaphragm deflates, signaling that the needle is in the epidural space

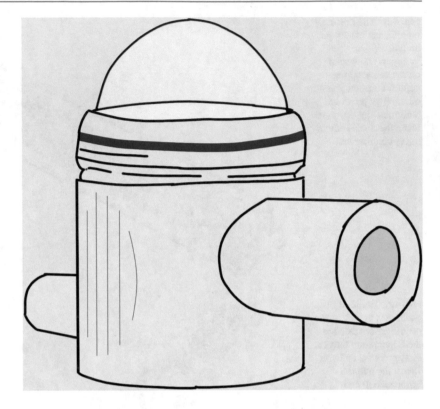

Fig. 4.8 LOR Indicator Syringe™: at the moment the needle reaches the epidural space, the bladder automatically releases the saline into the epidural space, and it is promptly shriveled, indicating a successful lumbar epidural puncture

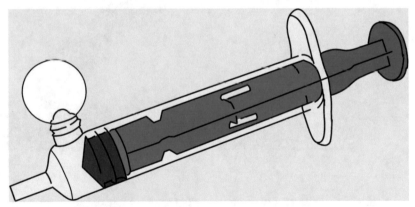

the balloon, connected to the epidural syringe, is filled with 3–5 mL of saline. Once the epidural needle is in the ligamentum flavum, the syringe is connected to the needle and the piston is pushed forward: doing so, the membrane is expanded owing to the resistance of ligament-induced pressure within the syringe, and forms a bladder which remains engorged. The needle is now slowly pushed forward (the needle retropulsion is forbidden) and at the moment the needle reaches the epidural space, and the bladder automatically

releases the saline into the epidural space and it is promptly shriveled, indicating a successful lumbar epidural puncture.

Other devices based on the loss of resistance principle are the EpiLong® Visual Pressure Control (VPC) syringe and the EpiFaith® syringe.

The EpiLong® VPC (Fig. 4.9) uses the Boyle-Mariotte law, according to which the product of gas volume and pressure is constant. Therefore, a capillary with a magnifying glass is integrated in the piston of the VPC. A pressure column, vis-

Fig. 4.9 The EpiLong®
VPC: A capillary with a
magnifying glass is
integrated in the piston
of the VPC. A pressure
column, visible in the
magnifying glass, is
built up under pressure.
If the VPC is connected
to the epidural needle
after skin puncture and
pressurized by pushing
the plunger forward, the
pressure column in the
capillary increases.
When the epidural space
is reached, the loss of
resistance becomes
visible by a drop of the
pressure column in the
magnifying glass of the
capillary

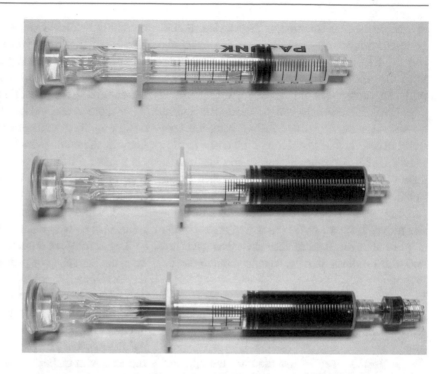

Fig. 4.10 The
EpiFaith® syringe: the
loss of the closed-system
pressure triggers a
warning signal, which is
the movement of the
rubber shaft

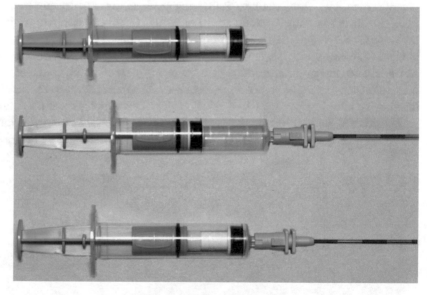

ible in the magnifying glass, is built up under
pressure. If the VPC is connected to the epidural
needle after skin puncture and pressurized by
pushing the plunger forward, the pressure column in the capillary increases. This remains visible as long as there is tissue pressure (resistance)
at the tip of the cannula. When the epidural space
is reached, the characteristic loss of resistance

becomes visible by a clearly recognizable drop
of the pressure column in the magnifying glass
of the capillary.

In the EpiFaith® syringe, the loss of closed-
system pressure triggers a warning signal, which
is the movement of the rubber shaft (Fig. 4.10).
The signal indicates that the needle tip has
entered a body cavity or that the system is oth-

erwise open. The function of this device should be tested prior to use by filling it with air occluding the exit port and then pushing the plunger until the color ring is covered: releasing the exit port the rubber should move forward rapidly. The EpiFaith® syringe can be used with liquid or air. After having filled the syringe, the epidural needle is inserted through the tissue until it reaches the ligamentum flavum. The stylet is then removed and the filled syringe is attached to the needle. Pushing the plunger slowly the pressure sensing (color ring) is activated. When the rubber moves forward or the color ring appears, this implies that the loss of resistance has occurred and the epidural needle advancement must be stopped.

4.1.4 Epidural Catheters

The materials used to manufacture the epidural catheter may vary from nylon to Teflon and are designed in the attempt to facilitate the ease of threading and to reduce the incidence of paresthesia and of intravascular cannulation (Fig. 4.11a). Material and design of an epidural catheter may also influence the catheter breakage, occlusion, kinking, or knotting.

In order to facilitate threading and increase the chance of successful insertion, many commercially available catheters are made of nylon blends with intermediate bending stiffness. Some nylon and polyurethane catheters have an inner stainless steel wire coil to increase rigidity, with fewer coils in the distal tip to impart flexibility.

A more recent advance in epidural catheter design is the development of wire-reinforced flexible catheters. Wire-reinforced flexible catheters have a thin outer wall and are reinforced with an inner wire spring that is loosely coiled in the distal tip, which altogether makes for a more flexible catheter compared to the non-wire-reinforced conventional catheters.

The rigidity of catheter materials may influence the incidence of paresthesia.

Soft-tipped, flexible catheters are commonly believed to result in fewer paresthesia because they may more easily change course as they encounter a nerve root or other obstacles in the epidural space. The paresthesia rate may also be reduced with catheters made from materials that soften at body temperature, such as polyurethane [21], or with the spring-wound polyurethane catheters [22, 23].

Catheter materials can also influence the incidence of intravascular cannulation. In general, softer, and in particular flexible, wire-reinforced polyurethane catheters are associated to a lower incidence of intravascular cannulation compared to conventional catheters [24].

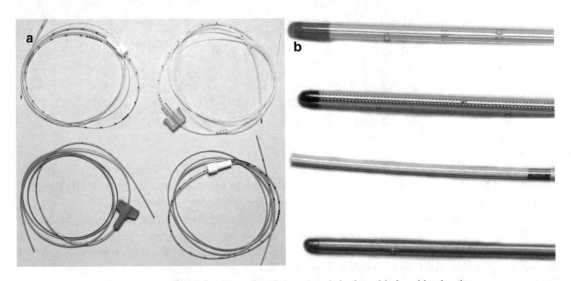

Fig. 4.11 (a) Epidural catheters. (b) Multiorifice, closed-tipped, and single end-hole epidural catheters

Catheter breakage also seems to be related to the mechanical properties of materials used. The materials with the lowest tensile strength are polyethylene and Teflon [25]. Polyurethane catheters may stretch more than 300% of their original length without breaking, whereas all other catheters broke before the elongation limit of the tensile testing machine [26].

The spring-wound polyurethane catheters stretch significantly more than the conventional non-wire-reinforced nylon catheters [27].

Catheter occlusion, kinking, and/or knotting may be associated with a number of factors, including the materials used to manufacture the catheter, the port configuration, and, in the case of wire-reinforced catheters, the method of attaching the inner wire coil to the surrounding coating. However other factors such as depth of insertion and method of catheter fixation to the skin may also play an important role.

Wire-reinforced catheters have better kink resistance, better flow characteristics, and improved patency when compared to non-wire-reinforced versions [28]. However, flexible catheters may be more difficult to remove and may be severely damaged during the removing procedure [29–31].

These features may be related to the type of catheter material (nylon, polyurethane, or a nylon-polyurethane blend) and to the technique used to attach the inner wire spring to the outer wall (integration of just the proximal and distal ends versus the entire length of the inner wire coil into the outer wall).

The position and number of catheter ports may affect the spread of analgesia, the incidence of paresthesia and intravascular cannulation, and the potential for a multicompartmental block (Fig. 4.11b). Multiorifice, closed-tipped catheters, when compared with single end-hole catheters, facilitate and improve the distribution of the solution in the epidural space and are significantly associated to better analgesia and satisfactory block [32–34]. They have the greater likelihood that aspiration of cerebrospinal fluid or blood can occur from one of the orifices in the event of a misplaced catheter, and diminished likelihood of orifice blockage by a clot or adjacent tissue [35].

In addition, the blunt-tipped multiport catheter is potentially less traumatic, reducing the likelihood of intravascular cannulation. However, a multiport catheter can result in a multicompartment block [36] and preferential efflux from a single or all ports based on the rate and pressure of the injected solution [37].

The incidence of paresthesia, venous cannulation, and reinsertion related to venipuncture seems to be less with the newer open-end, uniport spring-wound polyurethane catheters [38]. Multiple ports do not appear to improve the analgesic efficacy of the wire-reinforced flexible catheters [39].

An epidural catheter which is claimed to combine the benefits of the two different types of catheters is the so-called combined end-multiple lateral hole epidural catheter (CEMLH) [40] which has seven holes: one at the tip, and the others arranged circumferentially. The claimed advantages are that the end hole can recognize an inadvertent intravascular or subarachnoid insertion, the six lateral holes may allow the injection in the case that the end hole or one of the lateral holes are obstructed, and it may also provide a better distribution of the anesthetic solution.

Usually the epidural catheters have a length of 8–9 cm and are provided with markings to guide anesthetists as to the length left in the epidural space. However, depending on the manufacturer, the positions of these markings may vary, because the centimeter markings begin at different distances along the catheters. Many epidural catheters are transparent with a radiopaque line for ease of location in case of rupture.

4.1.5 Epidural Filters

Although may be unlikely especially in the very-short-term epidural catheterization in healthy patients, such as that for labor analgesia, microbial colonization of the epidural catheter may be a source of epidural infection. Microbial colonization could result from contamination of the infused fluid or the delivery system or from hematogenous seeding at the catheter tip, but the

Fig. 4.12 Flat filter
(fibrillary structure
1000× magnification)
(from [46] with
permission)

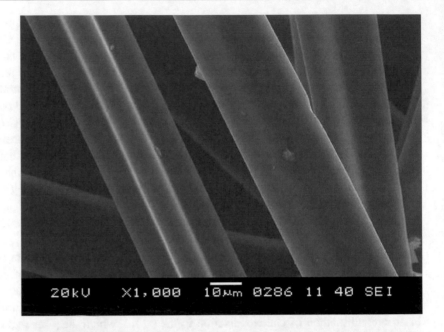

Fig. 4.13 Flat filter
(granular structure
5000× magnification)
(from [46] with
permission)

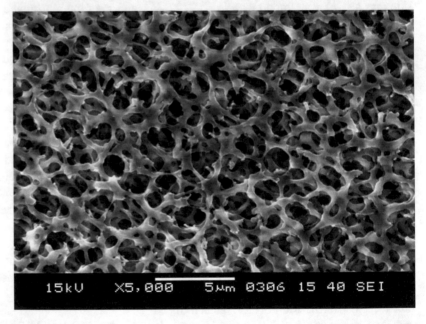

most important factor is the invasion of organisms present at the insertion site along the catheter track [41].

Bacterial filters have been deemed not to be needed in continuous epidural analgesia for healthy obstetric patients [42–44], but it seems reasonable to use them also in this low-risk setting, since positive epidural catheter tip cultures may occur despite the use of full aseptic and antiseptic precautions when the epidural filters have not been used [45].

However it should be remembered that adhering strictly to aseptic techniques is the most important factor in lowering the incidence of contamination.

Filters may have basically two kinds of structure, fibrillary and granular (Figs. 4.12 and 4.13), and can be made of polyvinyl chloride or cellulose acetate. In long-term epidural catheterization granular filters are more successful in the adhesion of dense bacteria suspension than the ones with fibria [46].

Epidural filters may be used to prevent foreign material from gaining access to the epidural space, although using epidural filters does not guarantee against the access of foreign materials that may be introduced before the interposition of the filter.

Some filters are made from hydrophilic supported membrane that allows two-way filtration and the ability to test the aspirate.

4.1.6   Connectors

Misconnections, such as between the intrathecal and intravenous lines, may be possible because the design of the devices is such that it is possible to inadvertently connect the wrong syringes and tubing and then deliver medication or fluids through an unintended and therefore wrong route. This is due to the multiple devices used for different routes of administration being able to connect to each other. The International Standards Organization (ISO) committee (ISO TC210 JWG4) has promoted the establishment and the implementation of a universal design specification for a non-Luer neuraxial connector (Figs. 4.14 and 4.15). The Joint Commission issued Sentinel Event Alert 53, in which they gave indications regarding managing the risk during the transition to new ISO tubing connector standards [47]. The new ISO 80369-6, NRFit connector for epidural regional anesthesia and other neuraxial application connectors, will no longer fit into ports other than the type for which they are intended, reducing the risk of misconnections between unrelated systems.

Changes to neuraxial connectors (NRFit) will follow the ISO standard 80369-6 design.

All medical devices which connect to the neuraxial route will eventually use the 80369-6 connector. Examples of devices affected include spinal needles, neuraxial/epidural syringes and syringe caps, manometers, Tuohy needles, epidural catheters, epidural filters, CSE kits (combined anesthesia), drawing-up filter needles, and drawing-up kwills, taps (two- or three-way taps) to be used with manometers. The market will produce, therefore, safer epidural connectors that will not connect epidural equipment (needles, epidural catheters, filters, and syringes) with intravenous Luer connectors or intravenous infusion spikes to reduce the risk of misconnection and the chance of injecting medication not intended for the epidural space.

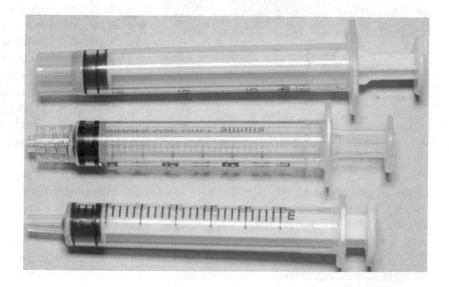

Fig. 4.14 From top to bottom: the ISO 80369-6, NRFit connector for epidural regional anesthesia, the standard Luer-Lock, and the standard Luer-Slip syringes

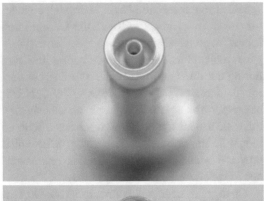

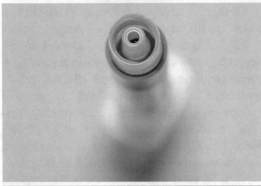

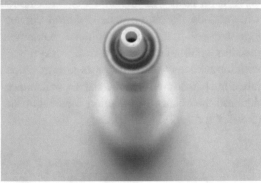

Fig. 4.15 From top to bottom: the ISO 80369-6, NRFit connector for epidural regional anesthesia, the standard Luer-Lock, and the standard Luer-Slip syringes (viewed from above)

4.2 Patient Position

Epidural block may be performed either in a lateral or in a sitting position (Fig. 4.16).

The patient position used for the insertion of epidural catheters for labor analgesia is generally related to the personal preference of the anesthesiologist and fetal condition or maternal factors rarely influence his/her choice. The preference of the physician is likely to be the position in which he (she) was taught to perform epidurals.

The favorite, routine position of the author of this book is the lateral one, and his choice is due to scientific and clinical evidence rather than how he learned the technique.

In the lateral position aortocaval compression is minimized and uteroplacental blood flow is optimized, since direct measurements of the uterine blood flow in the lateral position are associated with improved placental blood flow when compared to the sitting one [48]. In addition, continuous fetal heart rate monitoring is better obtained and maternal orthostatic hypotension is less likely in the lateral position.

With pregnancy, the obstruction of the inferior vena cava by the gravid uterus diverts blood into the vertebral venous system, which, when coupled with the expansion of intravascular volume, further engorges the epidural venous plexus.

These alterations in the epidural plexus can be minimized with changes in position. Changing from the supine recumbent position to the lateral position during pregnancy causes the engorged epidural venous plexus to return to nonpregnant size [49].

By contrast, in the upright and sitting positions, hydrostatic pressure within the lumbar epidural plexus increases.

For these reasons there is a lower incidence of epidural vein cannulation when the epidural block is performed in the lateral position as compared to the sitting position [50].

The effect of position on the hydrostatic pressure is not limited to the epidural plexus, but also affects the cerebrospinal fluid as well: in the sitting position there is an increased cerebrospinal fluid pressure which leads to dural bulging which may increase the chance of inadvertent dural puncture [51, 52].

Hence, the lateral position may decrease the possibility of inadvertent dural puncture.

However it is commonly believed that possible advantages of the sitting position are ease of maintenance of position, central position of the lumbar spines, and reduced distance from the skin to the epidural space [53, 54].

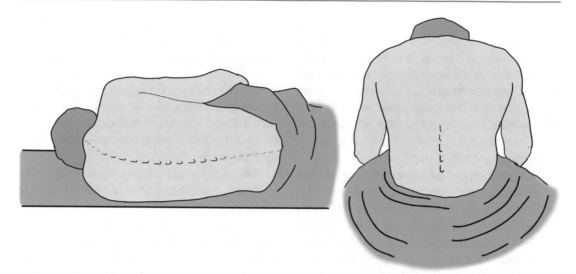

Fig. 4.16 Patient's position. Lateral position: the patient is placed in the lateral position with her back at the edge of the bed, legs drawn up to her abdomen, upper arm lying across her chest, and lower arm lying tight on the bed, with the head, resting on a pillow, flexed on the abdomen.

Sitting position: the patient is placed with her legs hanging over the side of the bed, her back towards the operator. The patient's arm is crossed or abandoned on the bent knees so as to retract the medial border of the scapulae away from the vertebral column

For these reasons the sitting position may be particularly preferred for obese women [55].

However obese parturients have a higher incidence of catheter displacement and this may be minimized by starting the block in the lateral position [53].

Although complications and maternal comfort during epidural insertion are not significantly affected by posture, the anesthesiologist should practice and be comfortable with neuraxial placement in the lateral position, as there are situations in which the sitting position cannot be used (fetal head entrapment, cord prolapse, presenting fetal limbs, or need to administer a blood patch). Furthermore, and most importantly, those practiced in using the lateral position can readily adapt to the sitting position, but the reverse does not apply [56].

4.2.1   Positioning the Patient

The parturient is placed in the lateral position with her back at the edge of the bed, legs drawn up to her abdomen, upper arm lying across her chest, and the lower arm lying tight on the bed, with the head, resting on a pillow, flexed on the abdomen.

Every effort is made to keep the spinous process of the vertebral column parallel to the table and the patient well flexed, so as to open the interspaces. In order to do that the shoulders and the iliac crest should be perpendicular to the table plane.

However, parturients may not flex their back very well, due to the gravid uterus.

Repeated or inappropriate efforts to improve dorsal flexion may result in bringing the upper shoulder forward towards the abdomen which rotates the spinous process of the vertebral column out of the parallel alignment with the bed surface and thus favoring the contact of the epidural needle on the vertebral bony arch during the attempt to reach the epidural space.

With regard to the sitting position, this is best assumed by placing the patient with her legs hanging over the side of the bed, her back towards the operator. The patient's arm is crossed or abandoned on the bent knees so as to retract the medial border of the scapulae away from the vertebral column. The assistant may allow the patient's forehead to rest on his/her chest.

For both the positions it is most important that the patient forcefully flexes the vertebral column to make the spinous processes more prominent and the intervertebral spaces wider. Flexion of the thighs on the spine does not necessarily cause flexion of the lumbar vertebrae. It is not sufficient to tell the patient when sitting to "bend well forwards", or when lying down, to "draw your knees up to your chin." A better position results from instructions such as "try to arch your back like a cat" or with a fingertip on the lumbar area, "I want you to push this part of your back."

Independently of the patient's chosen position, the epidural anesthesia tray and all the materials necessary for the procedure must be previously placed on a cart at the disposal of the operator. The cart is placed conveniently close to the back of the patient and to the right side of the operator (unless he/she is left-handed, and in this case it will be placed on the left side).

4.3 Landmarks Identification

4.3.1 Manual Palpation

Before scrubbing, the physician should survey the back and select the most appropriate interspinous space. The midline should be identified by palpating the vertebral spines transversely. On palpating the spinous processes through the skin it is determined that they are separated by a semisolid depression approximately 1 cm in length, called interspace, which can be easily palpated when the parturient is in the flexed position. However in pregnancy there is less space between the adjacent lumbar spinous process and several spinous processes and interspaces should be palpated to determine the widest interspace and the possible presence of scoliosis or vertebral column deviations.

The palpation via the iliac crests is the most frequently used technique to identify the level of the lumbar segments.

The intercristal line is a horizontal line drawn across the highest points of both the iliac crests in an anteroposterior lumbar radiography that was proposed by the French surgeon Thèodore Tuffier in 1901 as the landmark for the purpose of performing lumbar subarachnoid injection. In the general population, Tuffier's line (the imaginary transverse line connecting the tops of the iliac crests) intersects the spine anywhere between the inferior end plate of the L4 to the superior endplate of the L5 [57]. However full-term parturients undergo physical changes such as overlordosis, pelvis rotation to the long axis of the spinal column, and body weight increase and Tuffier's line may cross the vertebral column at the L3–L4 interspace rather than the L4–L5 interspace (Fig. 4.17).

Fig. 4.17 Tuffier's line (the imaginary transverse line connecting the tops of the iliac crests) intersects the spine anywhere between the inferior end plate of the L4 to the superior endplate of the L5, but in term parturients this line may cross the vertebral column at the L3–L4 interspace (red line)

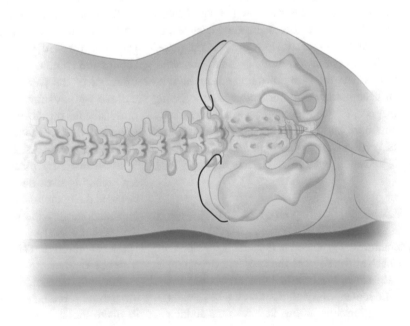

Vertebral levels are therefore more cephalad in parturient women as compared to non-parturient women, and this should be taken into account when performing an epidural block in term pregnant women [58].

Since the epidural space is widest at L2–L3 and the spinal cord usually ends at L1 but may extend to L2, mid-lumbar interspaces are usually selected for the puncture.

Unfortunately the accuracy of manual palpation is poor when it is eventually confirmed by ultrasounds [59, 60].

Theoretically the sitting position should improve the accuracy. In the sitting position, it is easier to eliminate the effect of lumbar lordosis and easy to determine the intercristal line as it gives a good grip by palpating both iliac crests. The distribution of body weight is even in the sitting position as compared to the lateral position where the patient is lying on an uneven surface. In the lateral position, the axis of the pelvic brim is deviated from the spine resulting in the variation in the position of Tuffier's line while the sitting position helps better to widen the lumbar interspaces and thus pushes Tuffier's line caudally to cross the L4–L5 space.

However, accuracy of the palpation is not improved by the use of the sitting position and is worsened by obesity [59, 61].

Fortunately, the precise level of puncture is a matter of indifference provided that it is below L2 (in the case of spinal or CSE anesthesia).

4.3.2   Ultrasound Identification

The first who used ultrasound (US) for facilitating lumbar puncture were Bogin and Stulin in 1971 [62]. Ten years after, Cork [63] described the use of US to localize the lumbar epidural space, and in 1992 Wallace [64] used indirect ultrasonographic guidance for epidural anesthesia in obese pregnant patients. US are now recommended for obstetric analgesia and anesthesia by the National Institute of Health and Clinical Excellence (NICE) [65].

A detailed description of the technique is beyond the scope of this book but a systematic approach to performing a lumbar ultrasound scan to aid neuraxial blocks has been described elsewhere [66].

Ultrasound can be used in two different ways to make the performance of an epidural block easier: one method is to use real-time ultrasound imaging, under sterile conditions, to observe the passage of the needle on the way to the epidural space, and this will be discussed in Chap. 7. In the second method (pre-procedure ultrasound) an initial ultrasound scan of the patient's lumbar area is performed to find the midline and the interspinous space in order to mark the position of each on the skin.

Advantages of the use of pre-procedure US for epidural placement include the help in visualizing the anatomy, selecting the correct intervertebral space, measuring the depth from the skin to the epidural space, and planning the angle of insertion for the epidural needle (Figs. 4.18 and 4.19). These advantages are even more helpful in morbidly obese parturients and with patients with altered anatomy, such as in the cases of previous lumbar spine surgery and kyphoscoliosis [67].

Nevertheless, it should be remembered that should the patient move after the external identification of the landmarks, the ultrasound suffers from the same problems of imprecision of marking/identification of the lumbar interspace as the manual palpation method.

Among the disadvantages, it should be said that lumbar spine ultrasound is not easy to learn, requires advanced training and instruction, and has a long learning curve, and the teaching methods are not standardized and may vary greatly from institution to institution and between countries [68]. Additional time is required before performing the block and this is an important issue in the obstetric analgesia setting.

The increased cost is also a factor that prevents the diffusion of this technique: to buy dedicated ultrasound machines may lead to a considerable increase of costs (for the machine itself and for training the physician staff), and may also be impractical for a busy unit [68].

An alternative to the standard US, the SpineNav3DTM technology has been recently developed to facilitate image interpretation of

Fig. 4.18 Pre-procedure ultrasound scan of the patient's lumbar area: paramedian sagittal oblique view of the L5–L3 junction. The sacrum is recognizable as a horizontal hyperechoic curvilinear structure, and the L5 lamina has the typical "sawtooth" appearance. The structures of the vertebral canal are visible through the intervening gap (courtesy of Dr. S Baglioni)

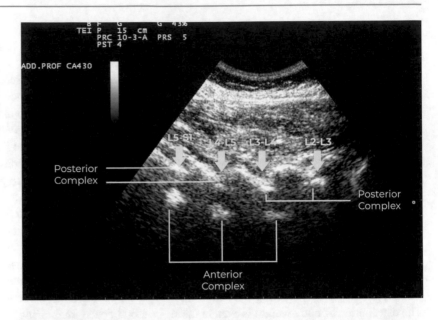

Fig. 4.19 Pre-procedure ultrasound scan of the patient's lumbar area: interspinous space transverse orientation (L3–L4) (courtesy of Dr. S Baglioni)

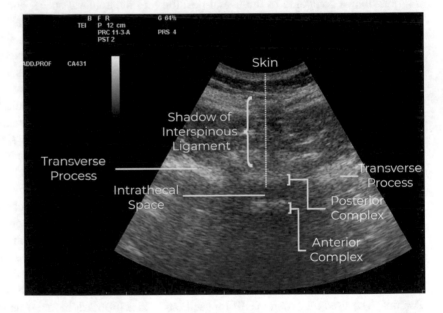

individual 2D lumbar spine scans by automating spinal bone landmark detection and depth measurements and providing a real-time assessment of scan plane orientation in 3D in a pocket-sized, battery-operated ultrasound instrument. This technology is able to provide some basic information such as detecting the bone landmarks and measuring the depth of the epidural space and is able to accurately predict the Tuohy needle depth to the epidural space [69] (Figs. 4.20 and 4.21).

Although pre-procedural US may be very useful and is suggested in difficult cases, at the present time, the ultrasound-guided technique to identify the landmarks for epidural and spinal blocks for obstetric patients should not routinely replace the traditional landmark and palpation technique, since large-scale studies are needed before advocating its widespread use. In fact, to date, there are no large randomized, blinded studies comparing epidural insertion with ultra-

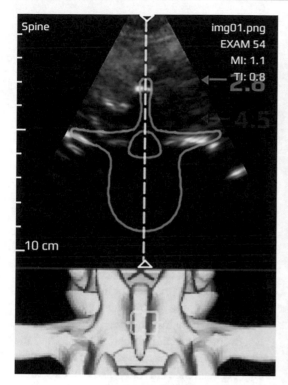

Fig. 4.20 Detecting the bone landmarks and measuring the depth of the epidural space with the SpineNav3DTM technology: midline indicator (white dotted line) along with a view of the 3D spine model. The blue number is the depth to the spinous process tip (in centimeter) (courtesy of Dr. S Baglioni)

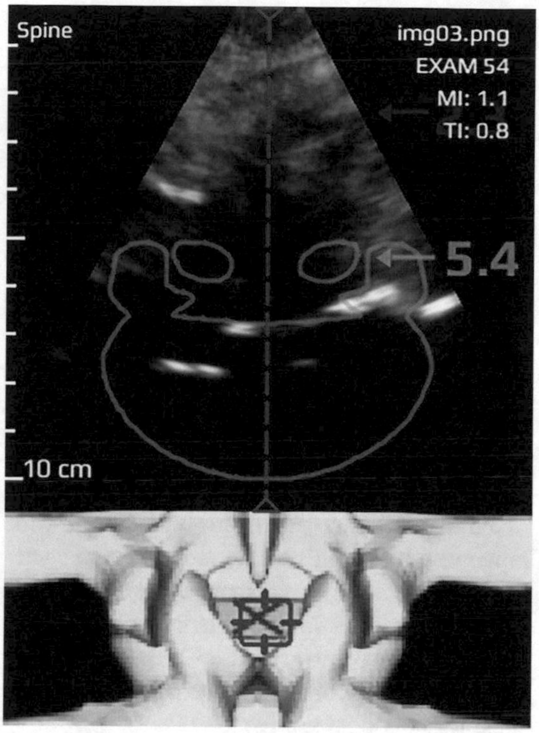

Fig. 4.21 Detecting the bone landmarks and measuring the depth of the epidural space with the SpineNav3DTM technology: midline indicator (red dotted line) along with a view of the 3D spine model. The orange number is the depth to the epidural space (in centimeter) (courtesy of Dr. S Baglioni)

sound to epidural insertion without ultrasound by an experienced anesthesiologist, in terms of speed of procedure, success rates, and complication rate. Indeed it is difficult to double-blind ultrasound studies, and this increases the risk of bias and limits the relevance and the impact of published results.

It should also be taken into account that the relationship with industry could influence the recommendations supported by studies promoting the widespread use of this technique.

In addition, although lumbar US does not directly scan the fetus, it is applied adjacent to the posterior aspect of the gravid uterus and prolonged scans have some potential to affect the fetus itself [70].

The traditional surface landmark-based technique is simple, safe, and effective in most patients. Instead, the utility of the ultrasound-guided approach is most evident in patients in whom technical difficulty is expected because of poor surface anatomic landmarks or distorted spinal anatomy.

4.4 Skin Disinfection

Handwashing remains the most crucial component of asepsis and gloves should not be regarded as a replacement for it [71].

The anesthesiologist wearing cap, facial mask, and sterile gloves applies the antiseptic solution over a wide area, including the iliac crest region down to the surface of the bed.

Surgical masks are advisable because of the increasing number of cases of postspinal meningitis, many of which result from contamination of the epidural or intrathecal space with pathogens from the operator's buccal mucosa [72].

While the applied antiseptic solution is drying, the anesthesia tray is checked for proper materials. Repeated application is unnecessary [73].

The ideal antiseptic agent should be effective against a wide range of microorganisms, have immediate onset of action, exert a long-term effect, not be inactivated by organic material such as blood, and have minimal adverse effects on the skin.

There is a wide range of practice among the anesthesiologists [74] and the commonly used antiseptic agents for epidural block include povidone-iodine and chlorhexidine gluconate. Both of these antiseptics are available as aqueous and alcoholic solutions.

Povidone-iodine is effective against a wide range of gram-positive and gram-negative bacteria, but one of the arguments against its use is the fact that its antibacterial activity is inhibited by blood and other organic materials. However this disadvantage should not be a very important issue for neuraxial techniques.

Compared to povidone-iodine, chlorhexidine has a more rapid, long-lasting, and superior bactericidal effect and it is effective against nearly all bacteria and yeasts. In addition, epidural catheters inserted following the use of chlorhexidine are six times less likely to be colonized than when povidone-iodine had been used [75–78].

The alcoholic solutions are the most effective and the recommended concentration is that of 2% chlorhexidine in 70% alcohol [79].

Although chlorhexidine is clearly superior to povidone iodine, adhesive arachnoiditis has been reported in obstetric patients after chlorhexidine in alcohol was mistakenly injected into the epidural space [80–82].

It has been suggested that alcohol, which constitutes the main component of chlorhexidine solutions, might be the causative neurotoxic agent [80], but there is some experimental evidence of neurotoxic effects of the simple aqueous chlorhexidine solutions too [83]. Some guidelines suggest that this remote potential for neurotoxicity is outweighed by the superiority in reducing surgical site infection [84–86], but it seems logical to advise the use of methods of skin application that minimize the risk of con-

tamination of the equipment and the gloves used by the physician, keeping the chlorhexidine solution separate from the block preparation trolley and, in all cases, to allow alcoholic solutions to dry following their application before starting the procedure, even if such a contamination may be more important when performing a spinal rather than an epidural block.

In addition to these considerations, it should also be noted that breastfed infants whose mothers had iodine overload applied for epidural anesthesia may have a risk for having postpartum elevated thyrotropin levels and requiring recall for retesting [87], while this feature is not observed when chlorhexidine 0.5% in 70% isopropanol has been used [88].

The most appropriate and safe antiseptic solution to use on the skin before epidural block unfortunately remains controversial [89].

Inadvertent injection of chlorhexidine into the epidural space is an anecdotical event; nevertheless it might occur, since chlorhexidine is a transparent liquid and may be mistakenly confused with other fluids present on the epidural tray.

Manufacturers of chlorhexidine still warn that this agent should not come into contact with meningeal/neural tissue; however both chlorhexidine and povidone-iodine have been shown to be cytotoxic to neuronal and Schwann cells, but chlorhexidine appears to be more toxic and to date no cases of arachnoiditis have been linked to the use of povidone-iodine [90].

4.5 Superficial Tissues' Local Anesthesia

Pain during the epidural procedure is very distressing to the parturient and fear of this may result in maternal reluctance to receive regional analgesia. Unfortunately also local anesthetic infiltration of the skin is described as painful.

A good strategy to minimize pain during injection is to perform the infiltration after having raised a superficial skin wheal, advancing the needle within the tissues very slowly, and also slowly injecting the anesthetic solution as the needle progresses.

Ideally the trajectory of the needle used for the infiltration of the superficial tissues should be the same as that which will subsequently make the Tuohy needle.

It is also important to allow an adequate length of time after skin infiltration and epidural procedure. For example, the minimum onset time after infiltration with 1% lidocaine is from 33 to 85 s in 95% of patients [91].

Some authors suggest that the use of epinephrine-containing lidocaine with the addition of bicarbonate may reduce superficial bleeding and pain on local anesthetic infiltration [92].

Recently needle-free injection systems have been introduced and used for local anesthesia prior to the neuraxial block for cesarean section (INJEX™ technology) [93]. These advanced systems work by forcing the liquid medication at an elevated speed through a small orifice without piercing the skin: the high-pressure fluid stream powers its way through the tissue resulting in a wider distribution of the medication especially in the least resistant tissues.

The advantages of using the needleless systems for delivery of local anesthetics are easy, with higher patient acceptance especially in cases of needle phobia. The main disadvantages are higher cost, the potential to frighten the patients due to the sudden noise produced, and the intense pressure sensations that occur upon delivery of the anesthetic.

4.5.1   Technique

The index finger and the middle finger of the non-dominant hand are placed parallel to the spine, indicating the interspace chosen ("landmark fingers"). They facilitate the proper placement of the needle in the center of the interspinous space, will indicate the landmark for the Tuohy needle insertion, and should be kept in place until the Tuohy needle reaches the next landmark, which is the ligamentum flavum (Fig. 4.22).

After having warned the patient of a pinprick, a small-gauge needle attached to a 5 mL disposable syringe containing the local anesthetic solution (such as 1 or 2% lidocaine) is inserted through the skin to make a wheal over the selected interspace and eventually gently inserted into the underlying tissues until the interspinous ligament, while the local anesthetic solution is slowly injected.

The angle of penetration should be the same as planned for the epidural needle.

Without moving the "landmark fingers," the epidural Tuohy needle will be inserted through the skin wheal previously made exactly in the middle of the interspace.

Aspiration is not necessary. It is very unlikely that a 22G or 25G needle may penetrate and stay in a very small, thin dermal blood vessels especially if the needle is advanced constantly, and, in all cases, the total amount of the local anesthetic to be used is far away from any toxicity.

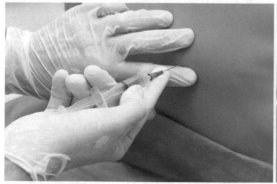 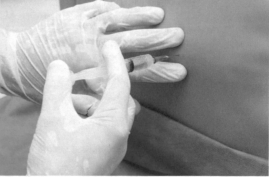

Fig. 4.22 Superficial tissues' local anesthesia: the index finger and the middle finger of the nondominant hand are placed parallel to the spine, indicating the interspace chosen ("landmark fingers"). They facilitate the proper placement of the needle in the center of the interspinous space and will indicate the landmark for the Tuohy needle insertion

Other authors prefer to mark the identified site of puncture with a mark using the thumbnail pressure or a dermographic pencil, to be used either for local anesthesia or for introduction of the Tuohy needle. However, in my personal opinion, any mark on the skin may not necessarily correspond to the previously identified landmark at the time the physician performs the epidural puncture if the patient moves, and this happens very often in laboring women.

References

1. Dogliotti AM. Trattato di Anestesia. Torino: UTET; 1935. p. 469.
2. Aburel E. L'anesthèsie locale (prolongèe) en obstètrique. Bullettin de la Società d'Obstètrique et Gynècologie de Paris. 1931;20:35–27.
3. Lemmon WT. A method for continuous spinal anesthesia. Ann Surg. 1940;111:141–4.
4. Huber RL. Hypodermic needle. US patent 2 409 979. October 22, 1946.
5. Tuohy EB. Continuous spinal anesthesia: its usefulness and technic involved. Anesthesiology. 1944;5:142–8.
6. Martinez Curbelo M. Anestesia peridural continua segmentaria con cateter ureteral utlizando la aguja de Tuohy caliber 16 con punta de Huber. La Havana: Reunion Anual de Cirujanos Cubanos; 1947.
7. Flowers CE, Hellman LM, Hingson RA. Continuous peridural anesthesia and analgesia for labor, delivery and cesarean section. Curr Res Anesth Anal. 1949;28:181–9.
8. Monoject [product data sheet]. St. Louis: Sherwood Medical, 1974; PD-222, 4.
9. Crawford OB, Ottsen P, Buckingham WW, et al. Peridural anesthesia in thoracic surgery: a review of 677 cases. Anesthesiology. 1951;12:73–84.
10. Benhardt AC, Jespersen K, Kodali BS. Anatomy of the epidural needle. SOAP 50th annual meeting, 9–15 May 2018, Miami, Poster S1B-3.
11. Poll JS. The story of the gauge. Anaesthesia. 2002;54:575–81.
12. Dunn SM, Steinberg RB, O'Sullivan PS, et al. A fractured epidural needle: case report and study. Anesth Analg. 1992;75:1050–2.
13. Russell R. The need for epidural wings. Anaesthesia. 2005;60:1048–9.
14. Patrick A, Miller C. More on epidural needle wings. Anaesthesia. 2006;61:405–6.
15. Kartal S, Kosem B, Kilinc H, et al. Comparison of Epidrum, Epi-Jet, and loss of resistance syringe technique for identifying the epidural space in obstetric patients. Niger J Clin Pract. 2017;20:992–7.
16. Duniec L, Nowakowski P, Sieczko J, et al. Comparison of the techniques for the identification of the epi-

dural space using the loss of resistance technique or an automated syringe. Anaesthesiol Intensive Ther. 2016;48:228–33.
17. Riley ET, Carvalho B. The Episure syringe: a novel loss of resistance syringe for locating the epidural space. Anesth Analg. 2007;105:1164–6.
18. Wantman A, Hancox N, Howell PR. Techniques for identifying the epidural space: a survey of practice among anesthetists in the UK. Anaesthesia. 2006;61:370–5.
19. Sawada A, Kii N, Yoshikawa Y, et al. Epidrum: a new device to identify the epidural space with an epidural Tuohy needle. J Anesth. 2012;26:292–5.
20. Xiaofeng L, E-er-dun W, Quing Y, et al. Clinical application of a novel developed pressure bladder indicator in lumbar epidural puncture. J Clin Anesth. 2015;27:543–5.
21. Bouman EA, Gramke HF, Wetzel N, et al. Evaluation of two different epidural catheters in clinical practice: narrowing down the incidence of paresthesia! Acta Anaesthesiol Belg. 2007;58:101–5.
22. Banwell BR, Morley-Forster P, Krause R. Decreased incidence of complications in parturients with the arrow (FlexTip Plus) epidural catheter. Can J Anaesth. 1998;45:370–2.
23. Terasako K. Reduced risk of intravascular catheterization with a soft epidural catheter. Acta Anaesthesiol Scand. 1999;43:240.
24. Mhyre JM, Greenfield ML, Tsen LC, et al. A systematic review of randomized controlled trials that evaluate strategies to avoid epidural vein cannulation during obstetric epidural catheter placement. Anesth Analg. 2009;108:1232–42.
25. Nishio I, Sekiguchi M, Aoyama Y, et al. Decreased tensile strength of an epidural catheter during its removal by grasping with a hemostat. Anesth Analg. 2011;93:210–2.
26. Ateş Y, Yücesoy CA, Unlü MA, et al. The mechanical properties of intact and traumatized epidural catheters. Anesth Analg. 2000;90:393–9.
27. Asai T, Yamamoto K, Hirose T, et al. Breakage of epidural catheters: a comparison of an arrow reinforced catheter and other nonreinforced catheters. Anesth Analg. 2001;92:246–8.
28. Chiu JW, Goh MH. An in vitro evaluation of epidural catheters: tensile strength and resistance to kinking. Ann Acad Med Singap. 1999;28:819–23.
29. Chiron B, de Serres TM, Fusciardi J, et al. Difficult removal of an arrow FlexTip Plus epidural catheter. Anesth Analg. 2008;107:1085–6.
30. Asai T, Sakai T, Murao K, et al. More difficulty in removing an arrow epidural catheter. Anesth Analg. 2006;102:1595–6.
31. Bastien JL, McCarroll MG, Everett LL. Uncoiling of arrow Flextip plus epidural catheter reinforcing wire during catheter removal: an unusual complication. Anesth Analg. 2004;98:554–5.
32. Michael S, Richmond MN, Birks RJ. A comparison between open-end (single hole) and closed-end (three lateral holes) epidural catheters. Complications

and quality of sensory blockade. Anaesthesia. 1989;44:578–80.

33. Collier CB, Gatt SP. Epidural catheters for obstetrics. Terminal hole or lateral eyes? Reg Anesth. 1994;19:378–85.

34. D'Angelo R, Foss ML, Livesay CH. A comparison of multiport and uniport epidural catheters in laboring patients. Anesth Analg. 1997;84:1276–9.

35. Segal S, Eappen S, Datta S. Superiority of multi-orifice over single-orifice epidural catheters for labor analgesia and cesarean delivery. J Clin Anesth. 1997;9:109–12.

36. Beck H, Brassow F, Doehn M, et al. Epidural catheters of the multi-orifice type: dangers and complications. Acta Anaesthesiol Scand. 1986;30:549–55.

37. Fegley AJ, Lerman J, Wissler R. Epidural multiorifice catheters function as single-orifice catheters: an *in vitro* study. Anesth Analg. 2008;107:1079–81.

38. Jaime F, Mandell GL, Vallejo MC, et al. Uniport soft-tip, open-ended catheters *versus* multiport firm-tipped close-ended catheters for epidural labor analgesia: a quality assurance study. J Clin Anesth. 2000;12:89–93.

39. Philip J, Sharma SK, Sparks TJ, et al. Randomized controlled trial of the clinical efficacy of multiport versus uniport wire-reinforced flexible catheters for labor epidural analgesia. Anesth Analg. 2018;2:537–44.

40. Eldor J. Combined end-multiple lateral holes epidural catheter. Reg Anesth. 1996;21:271–2.

41. Holt HM, Andersen SS, Andersen O. Infections following epidural catheterization. J Hosp Infect. 1995;30:253–60.

42. Abouleish E, Amortegui AJ, Taylor FH. Are bacterial filters needed in continuous epidural analgesia for obstetrics? Anesthesiology. 1977;46:351–4.

43. Yuan HB, Zuo Z, Yu KW, et al. Bacterial colonization of epidural catheters used for short-term postoperative analgesia. Anesthesiology. 2008;108:130–7.

44. Wong CA, Nathan N, Brown DL. Chapter 12: spinal, epidural, and caudal anesthesia: anatomy, physiology and technique. In: Clark V, Vand de Velde M, Fernando R, editors. Oxford textbook of obstetric anaesthesia. Oxford: Oxford University Press; 2016. p. 235.

45. Sahay M, Dahake S, Mendiratta DK, et al. Bacteriological profile of epidural catheters. JK Sci. 2010;12:23–6.

46. Sener A, Erkin Y, Sener A, et al. In vitro comparison of epidural bacteria filters permeability and screening scanning electron microscopy. Rev Bras Anestesiol. 2015;65:491–6.

47. Managing risk during transition to new ISO tubing connector standards, Sentinel Event Alert, The Joint Commission. 2014;(53).

48. Suonio S, Simpanen AL, Olkkonen H, et al. Effect of the left lateral recumbent position compared with the supine and upright positions on placental blood flow in normal late pregnancy. Ann Clin Res. 1976;8:22–6.

49. Hirabayashi Y, Shimizu R, Fukuda H, et al. Effects of the pregnant uterus on the extradural venous plexus in the supine and lateral positions, as determined by magnetic resonance imaging. Br J Anaesth. 1997;78:317–9.

50. Tsen LC. Neuraxial techniques for labor analgesia should be placed in the lateral position. Int J Obstet Anesth. 2008;17:146–52.

51. Hirasawa Y, Bashir WA, Smith FW, et al. Postural changes of the dural sac in the lumbar spines of asymptomatic individuals using positional stand-up magnetic resonance imaging. Spine. 2007;32:E136–40.

52. Carlson GD, Oliff HS, Gorden C, et al. Cerebral spinal fluid pressure: effects of body position and lumbar subarachnoid drainage in a canine model. Spine. 2003;28:119–22.

53. Hamilton CL, Riley ET, Cohen SE. Changes in the position of epidural catheters associated with patient movement. Anesthesiology. 1997;86:778–84.

54. Hamza J, Smida M, Benhamou D, et al. Parturient's posture during epidural puncture affects the distance from skin to epidural space. J Clin Anesth. 1995;7:1–4.

55. Vincent RD, Chestnut DH. Which position is more comfortable for the parturient during identification of the epidural space? Int J Obstet Anesth. 1991;1:9–11.

56. Stone PA, Kilpatrick WA, Thorburn J. Posture and epidural catheter insertion. Anaesthesia. 1990;45:920–3.

57. Snider KT, Kribs JW, Snider EJ, et al. Reliability of Tuffier's line as an anatomic landmark. Spine. 2008;33:E161–5.

58. Kim SH, Kim DY, Han JI, et al. Vertebral level of Tuffier's line measured by ultrasonography in parturients in the lateral decubitus position. Korean J Anesthesiol. 2014;67:181–5.

59. Parate LH, Manjunath B, Tejesh CA, et al. Inaccurate level of intervertebral space estimated by palpation: the ultrasonic revelation. Saudi J Anaesth. 2016;10:270–5.

60. Schlotterbeck H, Schaeffer R, Dow WA, et al. Ultrasonographic control of the puncture level for lumbar neuraxial block in obstetric anesthesia. Br J Anaesth. 2008;100:230–4.

61. Broadbent CR, Maxwell WB, Ferrie R, et al. Ability of anesthetists to identify a marked lumbar interspace. Anaesthesia. 2000;55:1106–26.

62. Bogin IN, Stulin ID. Application of the method of two-dimensional echospondylography for determining landmarks in lumbar punctures. Zh Nevropatol Psikhiatr Im S S Korsakova. 1971;71:1810–1.

63. Cork RC, Krye JJ, Vaughan RW. Ultrasonic localization of the lumbar epidural space. Anesthesiology. 1980;52:513–6.

64. Wallace DH, Currie JM, Gilstrap LC, et al. Indirect sonographic guidance in obese pregnant patients. Reg Anesth. 1992;17:233–6.

65. National Institute for Health and Clinical Excellence. Ultrasound-guided catheterization of the epidural space. London: National Institute for Health and Clinical Excellence; 2008. isbn. 1-84629-583-I.

66. Chin KJ, Karmakar MK, Peng P. Ultrasonography of the adult thoracic and lumbar spine for the central neuraxial blockade. Anesthesiology. 2011;114:1459–85.

67. Vallejo MC. Pre-procedure neuraxial ultrasound in obstetric anesthesia. J Anesth Perioper Med. 2017;5:85–91.

68. Margarido CB, Arzola C, Balki M, et al. Anesthesiologist' learning curves for ultrasound of the lumbar spine. Can J Anaesth. 2010;57:120–6.

69. Capogna G, Baglioni S, Milazzo V, et al. Accuracy of the SpineNav3DTM technology to measure the depth of epidural space: a comparison with the standard ultrasound technique in pregnant volunteers. Open J Anesth. 2018;8:113–22.

70. Nelson TR, Fowlkes JB, Abramowicz JS, et al. Ultrasound biosafety considerations for the practicing sonographer and sonologist. J Ultrasound Med. 2009;28:139–50.

71. Saloojee H, Steenhoff A. The health professional's role in preventing nosocomial infections. Postgrad Med J. 2001;77:16–9.

72. Schneeberger PM, Janssen M, Voss A. Alpha-hemolytic streptococci: a major pathogen of iatrogenic meningitis following lumbar puncture. Case reports and a review of the literature. Infection. 1996;24:29–35.

73. Malhotra S, Dharmadasa A, Yentis SM. One vs. two applications of chlorhexidine/ethanol for disinfecting the skin: implication for regional anaesthesia. Anaesthesia. 2011;66:574–8.

74. Bradbury CL, Hale B, Mather I, et al. Skin disinfection before spinal anaesthesia for caesarean section: a survey of UK practice. Int J Obstet Anesth. 2011;20:101–2.

75. Darouiche RO, Wall MJ, Itani KMF, et al. Chlorhexidine-alcohol versus povidone- iodine for surgical-site antisepsis. N Engl J Med. 2010;362:18–26.

76. Maki DG, Ringer M, Alvarado CJ. Prospective randomized trial of povidone-iodine, alcohol, and chlorhexidine for prevention of infection associated with central venous and arterial catheters. Lancet. 1991;338:339–43.

77. Sakuragi T, Yanagisawa K, Dan K. Bactericidal activity of skin disinfectants on methicillin-resistant Staphylococcus aureus. Anesth Analg. 1995;81:555–8.

78. Mimoz O, Karim A, Mercat A, et al. Chlorhexidine compared with povidone-iodine as skin preparation before blood culture. A randomized, controlled trial. Ann Intern Med. 1999;131:834–7.

79. Pratt RJ, Pellowe CM, Wilson JA, et al. Epic2: national evidence-based guidelines for preventing healthcare-associated infections in NHS hospitals in England. J Hosp Infect. 2007;65:S1–64.

80. Patle V. Arachnoiditis: alcohol or chlorhexidine? Anaesthesia. 2013;68:425.

81. Kocabas H, Salli A, Demir AH, et al. Comparison of phenol and alcohol neurolysis of tibial nerve motor branches to the gastrocnemius muscle for treatment of spastic foot after stroke: a randomized controlled pilot study. Eur J Phys Rehabil Med. 2010;46:5–10.

82. Miller B. Arachnoiditis: are we accusing the wrong agent(s)? Anaesthesia. 2013;68:423.

83. Weston-Hurst E. Adhesive arachnoiditis and vascular blockage caused by detergents and other chemical irritants: an experimental study. J Pathol Bacteriol. 1955;38:167–78.

84. Royal College of Anesthetists. Major complications of central neuraxial block in the United Kingdom. Report and findings of the 3rd National Audit Project of the Royal College of Anesthetists, 2009.

85. Horlocker TT, Birnbach DJ, Connis RT, et al. Practice advisory for the prevention, diagnosis, and management of infectious complications associated with neuraxial techniques. A report by the American Society of Anesthesiologists task force on infectious complications associated with neuraxial techniques. Anesthesiology. 2010;112:530–45.

86. Hebl JR. The importance and implications of aseptic techniques during regional anesthesia. RAPM. 2006;31:311–23.

87. Chanoine JP, Boulvain M, Bourdoux P, et al. Increased recall rate at screening for congenital hypothyroidism in breast fed infants born to iodine overloaded mothers. Arch Dis Child. 1988;63:1207–10.

88. Chanoine JP, Pardou A, Bourdoux P, et al. Withdrawal of iodinated disinfectants at delivery decreases the recall rate at neonatal screening for congenital hypothyroidism. Arch Dis Child. 1988;63:1297–8.

89. Lowings M, Muddanna A, O'Sullivan G. Arachnoiditis: time to return to povidone iodine-alcohol for skin preparation before neuraxial blockade? Anaesthesia. 2013;68:423–5.

90. Doan L, Piskoun B, Rosenberg AD, et al. In vitro antiseptic effects on viability of neuronal and Schwann cells. RAPM. 2012;37:131–8.

91. Almeida GP, Boos GL, Alencar TG, et al. Onset of 1% lidocaine for skin infiltrative anesthesia. Rev Bras Anestesiol. 2005;55:284–8.

92. Carvalho B, Fuller A, Brummel C, et al. Local infiltration of epinephrine-containing lidocaine with bicarbonate reduces superficial bleeding and pain during labor epidural catheter insertion: a randomized trial. IJOA. 2006;16:116–21.

93. Gozdemir M, Demircioglu RI, Karabayirli S, et al. A needle-free injection system (INJEX) with lidocaine for epidural needle insertion: a randomized controlled study. Pak J Med Sci. 2016;32:756–61.

Epidural Technique

These are the words used by Dogliotti [1] to describe his own loss-of-resistance technique to identify the epidural space: "When the needle has penetrated the ligamentum interspinous for a certain distance and before it has gone through the ligamenta subflava into the spinal canal one removes the trocar and attaches a syringe filled with physiological saline. When an attempt is made to inject this fluid a very great resistance is met with since the interspinous Ligamentum and the Ligamenta subflava are so dense. If they can be injected at all, it will be only after the employment of considerable force. This resistance is most certain evidence that the needle is still in the posterior fibers of these tissues. The following maneuvers are then carried out: the syringe is held in one hand the thumb of which applies a continued and uniform pressure to the piston. The other hand slowly advances the needle into the tissues and when it has traversed a few millimeters the hand which is holding it will suddenly note a diminution in the resistance to its passage which has previously been due to the tissues of the ligamenta subflava. At the same instant the injection fluid enters freely. This is certain, practical and unequivocal evidence that the point of the needle has pierced the Ligamenta subflava and is in the peridural space which offers no resistance to the flow of the injected fluid. As soon as this position has been recognized the needle should be left in the position which it now occupies for its point is in the peridural space; any attempt to advance it farther would entail the risk of penetrating the dura."

5.1 Loss-of-Resistance-to-Saline Technique

After having positioned the parturient, selected the interspace, and disinfected the skin accurate local anesthesia is made as discussed in Chap. 4.

The index finger and the middle finger of the nondominant hand are placed parallel to the spine, indicating the interspace chosen ("landmark fingers"). They facilitate the proper placement of the needle in the center of the interspinous space, will indicate the landmark for the Tuohy needle insertion, and should be kept in place until the Tuohy needle reaches the next landmark, which is the ligamentum flavum. Without moving the "landmark fingers," the epidural Tuohy needle is inserted through the skin wheal previously made exactly in the middle of the interspace (Fig. 5.1). The epidural needle is held with the palm of the hand resting on the hub, and the shaft of the needle between the fingers of the dominant hand (Fig. 5.2).

Electronic Supplementary Material The online version of this chapter (https://doi.org/10.1007/978-3-030-45332-9_5) contains supplementary material, which is available to authorized users.

Fig. 5.1 Without moving the "landmark fingers," the epidural Tuohy needle is inserted through the skin wheal previously made exactly in the middle of the interspace

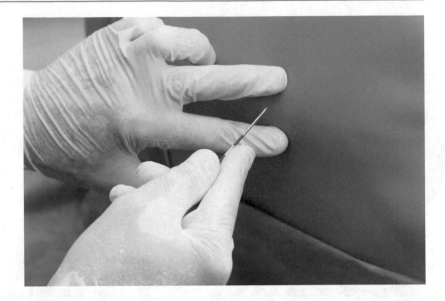

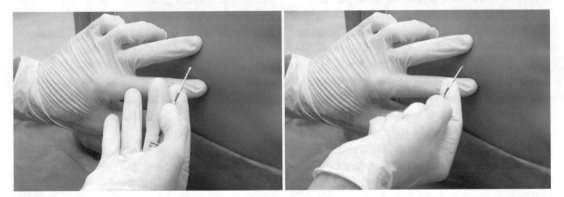

Fig. 5.2 The epidural needle is held with the palm of the hand resting on the hub, and the shaft of the needle between the fingers of the dominant hand

Once inserted into the skin, the epidural needle should be advanced with the bevel directed cephalad, taking care to remain in the midline (Fig. 5.3). The needle must be advanced very slowly but constantly, without any interruption, in order to be able to recognize the different densities of the underlying tissues (subcutaneous tissue, supraspinous and interspinous ligaments) during its advancement. As soon as it reaches the supraspinous ligament, a resistance is encountered due to the nature of the bevel, and the density of the ligament. The needle is then advanced through the loose interspinous ligament which offers much less resistance than the supraspinous ligament (often felt as a "no resistance feeling"

in the obstetric patient), until the point of the needle is felt to meet the third, and greater, point of resistance, the ligamentum flavum. This feeling of a greater increase of resistance is often associated with a "crunch" that indicates the initial penetration of the needle in the rear wall of the ligamentum flavum. Instead, if the resistance is absolute the bevel of the needle may be against the bony vertebral arch and any attempt to force the needle may result in pain for the patient due to periosteum stimulation. In this case the needle should be withdrawn, its angle of inclination checked, and the direction changed accordingly.

As soon as the point of the needle has engaged the ligamentum flavum, the advancement of the

Fig. 5.3 Once inserted into the skin, the epidural needle should be advanced taking care to remain in the midline

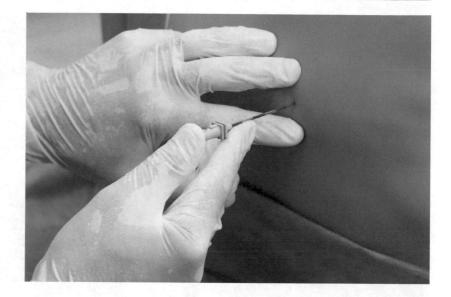

Fig. 5.4 As soon as the point of the needle has engaged the ligamentum flavum, the advancement of the needle is immediately stopped. The back of the left hand rests firmly against the patient's back to prevent advancement as the needle enters the epidural space with the hub of the needle grasped between the thumb and index fingers

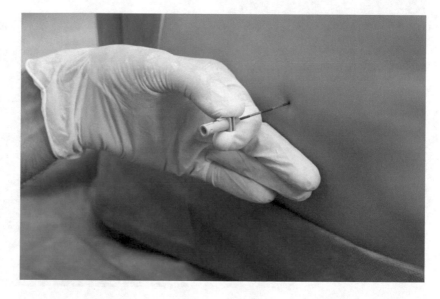

needle is immediately stopped, and the hands of the operator must change their initial position (Fig. 5.4). The back of the nondominant hand (usually the left hand) rests firmly against the patient's back to prevent advancement as the needle enters the epidural space with the hub of the needle grasped between the thumb and index fingers. The dominant hand (usually the right hand) removes the stylet (Fig. 5.5) and gently attaches to the needle a disposable 10 mL loss-of-resistance syringe containing no more than 5 mL of sterile saline solution.

Constant, unremitting, pressure is now exerted on the plunger of the syringe by the thumb of the dominant hand and since the content of the syringe (saline) is incompressible, the syringe and needle advance together solely by means of the pressure exerted by the operator on the plunger of the syringe (Fig. 5.6).

The physician should be totally concerned with pushing the piston, supporting the syringe, and interpreting the significance of changes in resistance to injection as the needle advances. Never advance the needle without simultaneous

Fig. 5.5 The right hand removes the stylet

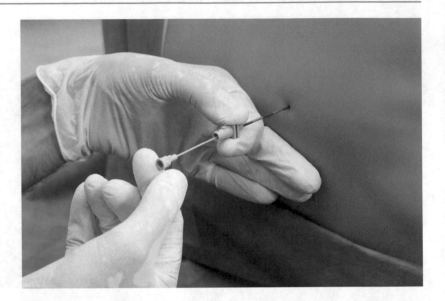

Fig. 5.6 The needle advances solely by means of the pressure exerted by the operator on the plunger of the syringe

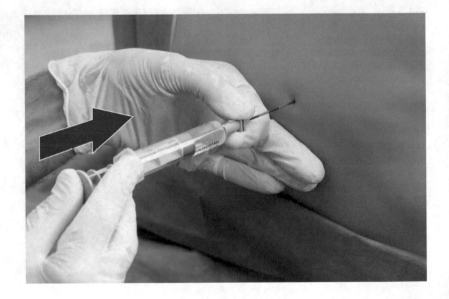

pressure on the plunger to tell you where you are: the needle is moved forward exclusively by the force exerted by the physician on the plunger of the syringe.

As long as the needle point is in the ligamentum flavum there is a great resistance to injection and the pressure exerted by the thumb on the plunger causes the advancement of the needle. The importance of moving the needle through the ligamentum flavum very slowly cannot be overemphasized. Several seconds should be allowed to advance the needle through the 3–5 mm thickness of the ligamentum.

As the point of the needle emerges from the ligamentum flavum into the epidural space, the resistance suddenly disappears and the advancement of the needle immediately stops, since the driving force exerted on the piston is discharged by the sudden entering of the liquid in the epidural space (Fig. 5.7). When practiced in this way, the loss-of-resistance technique is a "self-blocking system" and inadvertent dural puncture is unlikely.

Fig. 5.7 The point of the needle emerges from the ligamentum flavum into the epidural space. The resistance suddenly disappears and the advancement of the needle immediately stops, since the driving force exerted on the piston is discharged by the sudden entering of the liquid in the epidural space

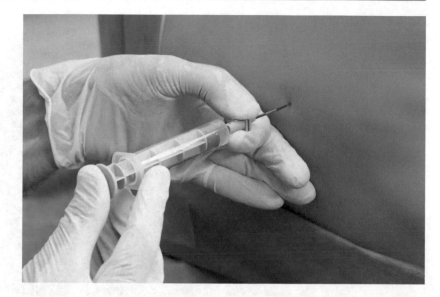

Fig. 5.8 When the epidural needle is positioned in the epidural space, the syringe is removed

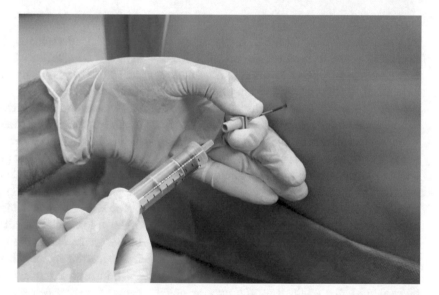

When the bevel is wholly within the epidural space, it is possible to inject saline with no resistance; therefore, if the operator experiences the sudden marked decrease in resistance, indicating the passage of the point of the needle through the ligament, but still feels that the injection is not completely free, the point of the needle may not be entirely within the epidural space and the needle should be advanced very slowly a few millimeters and the injection attempted again.

When the epidural needle is positioned in the epidural space, the syringe is removed (Fig. 5.8)

and the needle observed (Fig. 5.9) for the appearance of spinal fluid (sometimes a few drops of syringe solution may leak from the needle due to dural tenting) or blood.

5.2   False or Pseudo-Loss of Resistance

According to the original technique the needle should be entered until the dorsal aspect of the ligamentum flavum: in this way the very first

Fig. 5.9 The needle is observed for the appearance of spinal fluid or blood

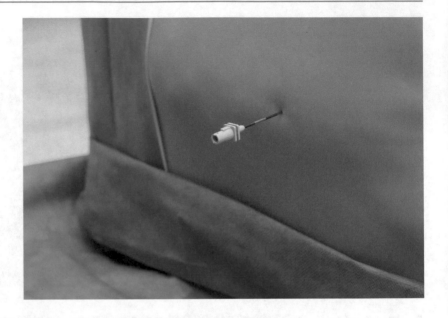

loss of resistance is, most likely, the right one. In clinical practice, however, the epidural needle is frequently introduced into the lumbar area to a depth of approximately 2–3 cm or somewhere between the soft tissues, due to the fear of accidental dural puncture.

In this case the needle is advanced slowly with only slight constant, unremitting pressure on the plunger of the syringe which allows the injection of a small amount of saline during the needle advancement within the tissues. Marked resistance to injection, allowing for greater pressure on the plunger, should be encountered when the needle point reaches the ligamentum flavum.

With this technique, difficulties in proper placement of the epidural needle may be noted especially initially, when there is little or no resistance to plunger pressure.

Most frequently, the false loss of resistance may occur superficial to the epidural space if the needle deviates from the midline, being of the side of the interspinous ligament, and enters the paravertebral muscles. In this case the relative loss of resistance may be mistaken for the more marked loss of resistance to the epidural space. Sometimes the injected solution may be pocketed under pressure between tissue planes and may drip back from there if the stylet is removed from the epidural needle. In addition if the needle enters the interspinous ligament at an oblique angle the needle tip will exit the ligament into the soft tissue on the opposite side with a loss of resistance-like feel.

When a doubtful increase in resistance is felt, the introduction of the needle must be stopped. If the needle has been inserted correctly into the ligamentum flavum, a slight pressure on the piston of the syringe will not determine any advancement of the piston itself. A further greater pressure on the piston will not again determine any advancement of the piston itself but will cause the advancement of the needle within the tissues corresponding to its progression into the ligamentum flavum.

If instead a modest pressure on the piston causes the advancement of the piston itself (corresponding to the leakage of a few drops of liquid from the needle) it is necessary to suspect that the resistance that was previously perceived was not that of the ligamentum flavum. To confirm this, it can be noted that the needle does not advance under the pressure of the piston operated by the physician. In this case it is most likely a false resistance, and the needle should be carefully and very slowly further advanced by a few millimeters and the maneuver repeated until a resistance to moderate pressure on the piston is obtained, suggesting that the needle could be in the ligamentum flavum.

5.3 Bone Contact

Although having an apparently correct insertion angle, the epidural needle may inadvertently hit a bone during its way in.

If the depth at which the needle is inserted is within the range of the vertebral arch and the physician has previously perceived the typical sensation of a "crunch" due to the initial insertion of the epidural needle within the ligamentum flavum, it can be assumed that the needle has encountered the vertebral lamina somewhere in the area where the ligamenta flava are inserted on the lamina (Fig. 5.10). In this case the needle is assumed to be very close to the full thickness of ligamentum flavum which can be reached by withdrawing the needle a few millimeters, and by redirecting and advancing it again by a few millimeters in the four directions (cranially, caudally, medially, and laterally, but usually and most frequently medially and cranially) until an increase of resistance (indicating that the bevel of the needle is in the ligamentum flavum) is perceived. The forward movement must be gentle, gradual, and continuous. Every advancement in any direction must be accompanied by a slight pressure applied to the syringe plunger to verify if there is any loss (false loss) or any increase (needle in the ligamentum flavum) in resistance.

If, instead, the depth at which the needle is inserted is not within the range of the vertebral arch, or if no increase in resistance (or "crunch") has been perceived before encountering the bone (Fig. 5.11), it should be remembered that the posterior surface of the lamina of a lumbar vertebra slopes downwards and backwards. If therefore the needle, slightly out of the median place, encounters bone at a shallow depth (Fig. 5.12), it is hitting the lower border of the lamina on which it impinges, whereas if the obstruction is deep, it is against the upper border. In these cases the position of the patient should be checked again and the needle must be reinserted with a different angle of inclination. In fact the parturient may not flex her back very well due to her protuberant abdomen, and with repeated efforts to improve flexion or with her inadvertent, involuntary movements during the procedure she may succeed only in bringing the upper shoulder forward towards the abdomen which rotates the spinal process of the vertebral column out of parallel alignment with the midline (and the bed surface): in this way the vertebral arch rotates on the midline and almost unavoidably the needle, introduced in the midline, hits it. For this reason in the case of bone contact the first thing to do is to check once again the correct position of the patient.

Fig. 5.10 The needle has encountered the vertebral lamina somewhere in the area where the ligamenta flava are inserted on the lamina

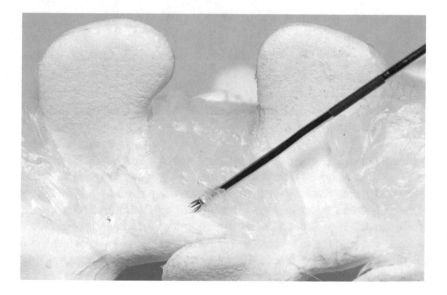

Fig. 5.11 The needle encounters the bone deeply (border of the lamina)

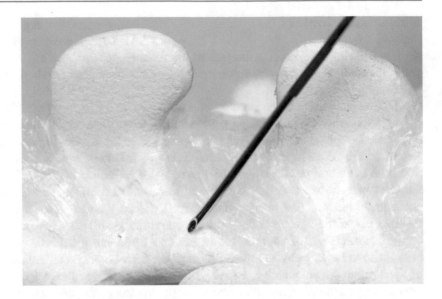

Fig. 5.12 The needle encounters the bone superficially (spinous process)

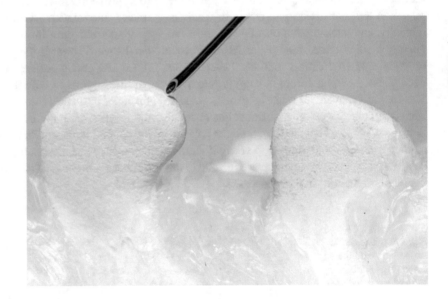

5.4 Observation and Aspiration of the Needle

Immediately after entering the epidural space the styled is removed (Fig. 5.9) and the needle observed for any leakage of fluid. Aspiration is then performed possibly with a small syringe since suction is greater with a small rather than a large one and therefore cerebrospinal fluid or blood are more easily detected if the dura or a vein has been inadvertently punctured.

If blood is aspirated it is best to abandon and repeat the procedure.

It is very easy to identify a significant free flow of warm fluid from the Tuohy needle as the cerebrospinal fluid. However, it is not uncommon to observe a small amount of clear fluid dripping from the Tuohy needle (or the epidural catheter) during uncomplicated insertion using a saline loss-of-resistance technique. Usually a few drops of liquid from the Tuohy needle are due to dural tenting that may cause a fluid reflux through the needle, especially if a large quantity of saline has been previously injected too rapidly and the back of the patient is extremely flexed. Following a large volume of saline into the epidural space, there is a temporary buildup of local epidural pressure, causing the solution to reflux briskly through the hub of the needle. Usually dripping due to fluid reflux ceases within 30–60 s; nevertheless, sometimes it may be difficult to distinguish between inadvertent dural puncture with leakage of cerebrospinal fluid (CSF) and dripping of saline from the epidural needle (or catheter).

Several techniques to distinguish between CSF and saline have been proposed, including testing for the presence of protein or glucose, temperature, pH, and changes in turbidity when mixed with thiopental. Glucose and pH tests are the most sensitive (<95%) [2]. Bedside glucometers and urine pH test strips or pH test papers (the pH value of CSF is between 7.317 and 7.324, and the pH value of saline is 7.0) are generally available on wards where obstetric epidurals are performed. Measurement of glucose or pH represents a sufficiently reliable, quick, and simple method to determine unintentional dural puncture if uncertainty exists. The difference in glucose concentration between epidural needle leakage (effectively zero) and CSF (significantly >zero; cerebrospinal fluid has a glucose content of >0.45 g.L) suggests that semiquantitative or even qualitative detection is adequate [3, 4].

However no single test is 100% reliable, so the physician should be familiar with various physicochemical tests since sometimes more than one test may be necessary to correctly identify the nature of the liquid [5]. If serious doubt exists about the correct placement of the needle it is best to restart the procedure and choose a new puncture site.

5.5   Rebound Test and Partially Inserted Bevel of the Needle in the Epidural Space

After negative aspiration for blood or cerebrospinal fluid, proper placement of the needle may be further checked with the air or rebound test.

A very small amount of air (1–1.5 mL) is drawn into the loss-of-resistance syringe and attached to the needle and the plunger of the syringe is tapped sharply. A positive test results when the syringe collapses and does not refill at all, or only refills 0.1–0.2 mL.

This rapid injection of a very few millimeters of air, mixed with the previously injected liquid already in the epidural space, may occasionally result in small air-water bubbles escaping from the hub of the needle. If this occurs, it may be considered another indirect sign of confirmation that the epidural needle is in the right place.

When the plunger rebounds, a partially inserted bevel of the needle in the epidural space could be suspected. The epidural needle should be cautiously advanced another millimeter, checked by pushing on the barrel of the reattached syringe filled with saline, and, after the complete and clear collapse of the piston (indicating the complete entry into the epidural space), the test should be repeated.

When the test is performed during a uterine contraction, a false-negative test may result.

A partially inserted bevel of the needle in the epidural space may also be the cause of a difficult or impossible insertion of the epidural catheter.

5.6   Loss of Resistance to Air

Fluid is incompressible and consequently the transition from complete resistance to loss of resistance is immediate and convincing. Air is compressible, so it is a less ideal physical agent than fluid, but it was introduced and deemed a good alternative to the loss of resistance to saline in the past, when the only syringes available were the reusable syringes made of glass, and the occurrence of the "sticky syringe" phenomenon was high enough to let physicians think about an alternative.

This occurred when the fluid dried from inside the syringe and left behind sticky residue, which basically "glued" the plunger to the barrel. Even though the syringe was usually rinsed with cleaning solvent after a sample injection, if the sample contained "sticky" material, not all of it may have got rinsed out. If this happened, and the liquid dried, the remaining residue bound the plunger to the barrel.

The adoption of an air-filled system appeared at that time a reasonable compromise.

Until the 1970s syringes were made of glass and were non-disposable, but nowadays with the widespread usage of the specifically designed plastic low-resistance syringes, the initial reason to use air is less convincing, and there is a trend towards a switch from air to saline [6].

The procedure and position of the hands are exactly the same as for a fluid-filled system. The only difference lies in the way the plunger of the syringe is compressed by the thumb of the dominant hand of the operator. Instead of continuous, unremitting pressure on the plunger, pressure is intermittent, alternating very rapid compressions and releases of the plunger, allowing the cushion of air to confer a series of rebounding oscillations to the plunger (Fig. 5.13). Never advance the needle without simultaneously applying these compressions to the plunger of the syringe. As soon as the needle passes the ligamentum flavum into the epidural space the plunger snaps forward as the cushion of air empties itself into the epidural space.

The proponents of using air claim that the use of saline may cause "confusion" with cerebrospinal fluid in the case of inadvertent dural puncture or reflux of cerebrospinal fluid due to dural tenting. This may be even more important with the needle-through-needle combined epidural spinal (CSE) technique (see Chap. 7). However there is no difference in the failure rate of spinal analgesia or efficacy of the epidural catheter function when using either air or saline in the loss-of-resistance technique for CSE labor analgesia [7].

In addition, in the case of dural tenting only a few drops of liquid are observed and aspiration is negative. Temperature, glucose, protein, and pH may be useful identifiers at the time of identifying the nature of a liquid coming from the needle [8].

The potential disadvantages of using air include partial block, increased incidence of accidental dural puncture, greater difficulty of epidural catheter insertion, higher rate of intravascular catheter insertion paresthesia, and risk of pneumocephalus [9, 10]. However, of these potential disadvantages only an increased risk of unblocked segments but no differences in the ability to locate the epidural space were reported in the meta-analysis [11, 12].

No consensus exists as to which technique is superior, and individual physicians currently use the technique with which they are most comfortable or that they were taught. There are, however, numerous case reports of severe complications associated with the use of air, which include pneumocephalus, spinal cord and nerve

Fig. 5.13 Loss of resistance to air. The pressure on the plunger is intermittent, allowing the cushion of air to confer a series of rebounding oscillations

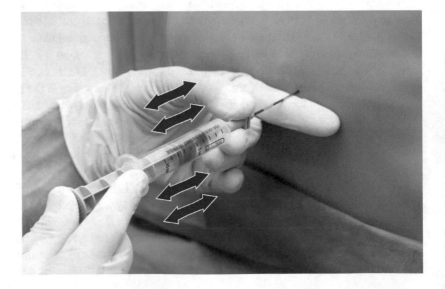

root compression, retroperitoneal air, subcutaneous emphysema, and venous air embolism [13]. These very rare but important potential complications associated with the use of air may outweigh the claimed benefits of its use.

However, it should be realized that the loss-of-resistance techniques to air and saline are two different techniques which every anesthesiologist should be familiar with, as early as possible, because any switch will signify a new learning curve.

5.7 Techniques Based on Epidural Negative Pressure

The "hanging-drop" technique is the main method based on the epidural negative pressure. This technique involves placing a drop of fluid into the hub of a winged epidural needle that has been inserted into the ligamentum flavum. The wings of the needle are grasped with the thumbs and index fingers and the operator's hands are steadied by the midline, ring, and little fingers resting on the patient's back as shown in Fig. 5.14. While the drop is watched constantly, the needle is slowly and continuously advanced. As soon as the ligamentum flavum is pierced and the bevel enters the epidural space, the drop is

suddenly sucked into the needle as if by a negative pressure in the epidural space.

This technique, therefore, relies on the aspiration of a small volume of fluid from the hub of the needle as the pressure at the tip decreases below atmospheric level upon entry into the epidural space. For this reason it is used for cervical and thoracic epidural blocks, where a negative pressure in the epidural space may be present, especially in the sitting patient and during inspiration, since inspiratory movements transmit a further increment in negative pressure to the epidural space [14].

In the lumbar epidural space there is no naturally occurring negative pressure and the negative pressure, occasionally recorded, is an artifact resulting from bulging of the ligamentum flavum in advance of the needle with its rapid return to the resting position once perforated [15]. In addition, in pregnancy and during labor the epidural space pressure is well above the atmospheric values, ranging from 4 up to 30 mmHg [16, 17].

I therefore perfectly agree with Prof. Bromage's words that "it is illogical to use the hanging drop test in the lumbar region and the technique should be confined to thoracic and cervicothoracic punctures" [18]. I would also like to say that this applies not only to the hanging-drop technique, but also to any other technique based on epidural negative pressure, such as epidural

Fig. 5.14 The "hanging-drop" technique. This technique uses the negative epidural pressure as a marker of finding the epidural space by placing a drop of saline on the hub of the advancing needle

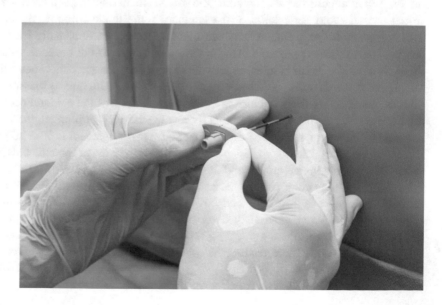

balloons or similar devices (see Chap. 4), since there is no rationale to use them in the obstetric patient and for lumbar epidural block.

5.8 Paramedian Approach

This approach has been specifically thought of for the middle thoracic region, where the obliquity of the spinous process is extreme. Although the paramedian approach is not commonly used in the obstetric patient, it may be used as an alternative to the midline approach when the introduction of the needle through the interspace is deemed difficult, or in the case of patients who are difficult to position.

The different angle of penetration of the needle in the epidural space may be the reason for the technical advantages advocated for this approach, which include a small risk of accidental perforation of the dura mater, no tenting of the dura by the tip of the catheter, and the promotion of a straight course cephalad in the near midline for the epidural catheter [19].

Typical features of this approach include a larger target through the interlaminar space as well as the avoidance of the puncture of the supraspinous and interspinous ligaments.

Local anesthesia is obtained by making a 2 cm wheal lateral to the midline, and infiltrating the subcutaneous tissues, including the paraspinal muscles and periosteum of the laminae. This injection not only aims to produce analgesia, but it also serves to make a path for the epidural needle. The latter is inserted into the skin and directed towards the medial extremity of the lamina. As soon as this structure is contacted, the needle is gently maneuvered so that its bevel reaches the superior surface of the lamina and therefore engages the tough ligamentum flavum. The stylet is then removed and the syringe filled with saline is connected to the hub of the needle. The needle is then advanced slowly and constantly in the way previously described in the paragraph on midline approach, until sudden lack of resistance indicates that the epidural space has been entered.

5.9 Forces Involved During Needle Insertion

A complete description of forces involved during needle insertion is complex. In particular, there is interplay between the reaction forces from the needle shaft in tissue versus the reaction forces from the plunger of the syringe. The complex needle insertion forces include tip/cutting forces, shaft friction, and non-axial forces and torques. The plunger force includes the needle orifice/tissue interface, syringe friction, syringe leakage, and saline compression. It is extremely difficult to accurately quantify these minute forces and therefore the measured resultant insertion pressure may represent a good surrogate.

Pressure increases as the needle passes skin, subcutaneous fat, and muscle.

The average maximal pressure observed when the needle perforates the ligamentum flavum ranges from 370 to 500 mmHg, corresponding to 4.9–6.6 Newton cm^2 (N), and is scarcely influenced by the parturient's body mass index [20, 21] (Fig. 5.15).

When the needle enters the epidural space, an exponential decrease in pressure is observed. The pressure present in the lumbar epidural space when no fluid is injected is approximately or slightly above the atmospheric pressure, but in the pregnant patient it is higher, ranging from 14 to 30 mmHg [22]. After a bolus of 10 mL of local anesthetic solution, the epidural space pressure increases transiently from 208 to 300 mmHg to return to the baseline values in 10 min [23]. In pregnant patients, when using a continuous pressure technique to measure the force pressure at the tip of the epidural needle and the pressure on the syringe plunger, the flow rate at the interspinous ligament is 60 ± 30 mm^3/s which is significantly larger than the flow rate in the ligamentum flavum at 12 ± 13 mm^3/s. The average force is also significantly larger in the ligamentum flavum (5.0 ± 3.0 N) than in the interspinous ligament (2.0 ± 1.4 N) despite the lower flow. The maximum force applied is 6.0 ± 3.0 N in the ligamentum flavum, significantly larger than in the interspinous ligament at 4.6 ± 1.3 N [24].

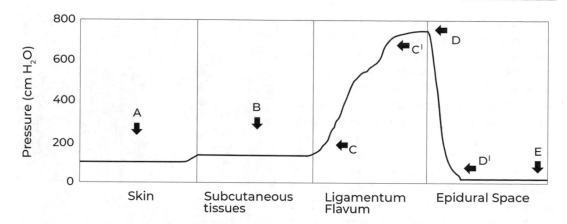

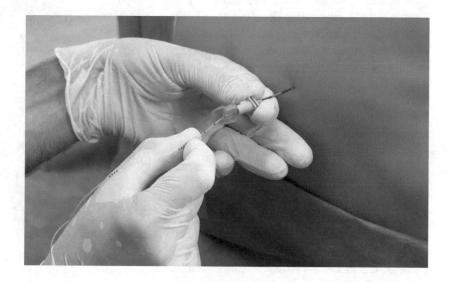

Fig. 5.15 Variations of pressure at the tip of the needle as it passes through the different tissues: the skin (**a**), the subcutaneous fat and muscle tissues (**b**), the ligamentum flavum (**c**), and finally the epidural space (**e**). Point (**d**) indicates the entrance to the epidural space. Arrow (**e**) indicates the end-residual pressures after 5 s of point (**d'**) (from [20] with permission)

Fig. 5.16 The epidural catheter is advanced through the needle

5.10 Catheter Insertion, Needle Removal, and Catheter Fixation

Once the needle is in place, the epidural catheter is advanced through the needle by the dominant hand while the back of the nondominant hand (usually the left hand) keeps resting firmly against the patient's back with the hub of the needle grasped between the thumb and index fingers (Fig. 5.16).

To increase the likelihood of cranial progression of the epidural catheter the beveled edge of the epidural needle may be oriented cranially, even if approximately only half of epidural catheters advanced into the lumbar epidural space through a cephalad-directed Tuohy needle reach the intended cranial level [25]. The parturient should be warned that sometimes she might feel an "intense tingle" in her hip or leg when the catheter is advanced a few centimeters beyond the bevel. Such paresthesia may occur when the epidural catheter contacts a spinal nerve root, depending on the type and on the material of the catheter, on the needle position (midline, paramedian), and on the epidural anatomy of the patient. To reduce the likelihood of paresthesias and inadvertent vascular puncture the patient should be asked to take a deep breath, in order to expand the epidural space, just immediately before and during the initial insertion of the epidural catheter [26]. The risk of intravascular placement of a lumbar epidural catheter in pregnancy may be reduced with the lateral patient position, fluid predistension (injection of 5 mL of saline in the epidural space before introducing the catheter), use of single-orifice and/or wire-embedded polyurethane epidural catheters, and limiting the depth of catheter insertion to 6 cm or less [27].

Sometimes difficulty is encountered in passing the catheter beyond the tip of the needle. This may be due to partial rather than complete entry of the bevel of the needle into the epidural space, or may indicate that the needle is not in the epidural space, having been inserted superficially into the ligamentum flavum. In the first case the needle should be very carefully and slowly advanced for 1–2 mm, and in the second case repositioned.

Occasionally after having advanced the catheter for 1–2 cm an obstruction is met. In this case its tip may have impinged on a fat pad or vessel, or the pedicle of vertebra above the injection site. In such cases, gently twisting the catheter on its axis will often change the position of its point so that it can be further advanced without difficulty. Withdrawing the catheter through the needle once its tip has passed into the epidural space may lead to the catheter shearing off, even if today most Tuohy needles are made with a rounded blunt bevel, and therefore this maneuver is not advisable or in any case should be performed very cautiously.

Before and after removing the needle, the catheter should be aspirated with a 2 or 5 mL empty syringe in order to detect blood and cerebrospinal fluid which are, respectively, signs of accidental intravascular and subarachnoid placement of the catheter (Fig. 5.17).

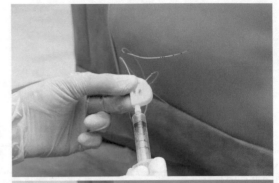
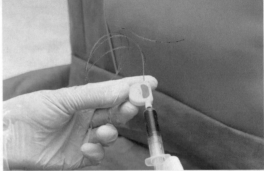
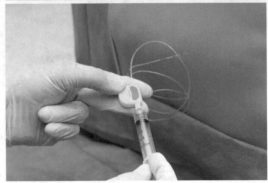

Fig. 5.17 Aspiration of the epidural catheter

If blood or blood-tinged fluid is aspirated, the catheter should be withdrawn an additional 1 cm and aspiration repeated. If no blood or CSF can be aspirated the syringe is disconnected and 1 mL of air or saline is injected to dislodge any tissue that may be against the tip of the catheter. Then, another attempt is made at aspiration. If again nothing is aspirated, a further precaution is taken: the syringe is detached and the end of the catheter is placed below the level of the spinal column: if it is in the subarachnoid space, fluid will drip out.

In all cases, even after a negative aspiration test, it is advisable to routinely make the additional maneuver to place the end of the epidural catheter below the plane of the bed of the patient and observe for the passive return of blood or cerebrospinal fluid.

After a negative aspiration test, the needle is removed. This is an important maneuver since the catheter may be dislodged from the epidural space while removing the needle. The catheter is grasped 1–2 cm distal to the hub of the needle by the thumb and the index finger of the dominant hand while the thumb and the index finger of the other hand pull the needle out of the back of the patient. The dominant hand should attempt to advance the catheter while the nondominant is pulling out the catheter (Fig. 5.18). At the end of the procedure, the catheter distance marks are checked and the catheter is properly positioned and aspirated again. Placement of the catheter more than 5 cm in the lumbar epidural space may be associated with a higher incidence of catheter

deviation into the intervertebral foramen causing unilateral block, and a greater likelihood of the tip entering an epidural blood vessel, while too little catheter length insertion predisposes the catheter to falling out [28].

When a catheter is pushed into the foramen against resistance, the catheter penetrates the areolar tissue and may deviate in the paravertebral area [29] and such a deviation is more likely with stiff catheters and less likely with soft, spiral-type catheters with an internal coil [30].

Epidurography and anatomical studies suggest that the most appropriate length that an epidural catheter should be left in the epidural space should lie between 2 and 5 cm [31, 32].

The catheter is then secured with tape and adhesive dressings, and used for the intended purpose. The ideal method of fixing catheters would encompass the optimal security of the catheter, ease of inspection, and maintenance of sterility at the site of insertion. Not only must an application function in dry conditions, but it must retain this

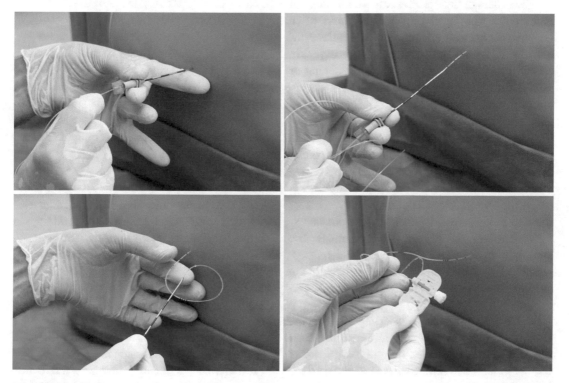

Fig. 5.18 Epidural catheter removal: the right hand should attempt to advance the catheter while the left is pulling out the catheter

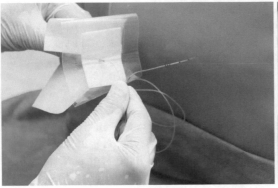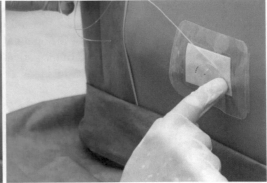

Fig. 5.19 Epidural catheter fixation

efficacy after exposure to blood, perspiration, and epidural solution (Fig. 5.19).

An adequate fixing of the epidural catheter should not be underestimated, because the percentage of epidural catheter dislodgment under adhesive dressing may be up to 16% [33] and unfortunately, despite the availability of a variety of catheter fixation devices, the problem of catheter displacement still persists.

The causes of the epidural catheters falling out include dragging on the epidural catheters when the patients are sitting or moving while the catheters are fixed to the shoulders, sweating, skin reaction to the dressing used causing itching or blister formation, inattentive movement during nursing, parturients' movements during labor and delivery, and so on.

The catheter can exit the epidural space via an intervertebral foramen giving rise to a patchy or unilateral block. Alternatively, it may retract into the soft tissues of the back, resulting in failure of analgesia. Fortunately, the movement of the catheter at the skin surface does not necessarily translate to migration of the catheter tip, but suggests that it may have become displaced. Notable migration of the epidural catheter at the skin surface may occur in more than 40% of parturients [34].

If the epidural catheter is firmly taped to the skin while the patient is still in the sitting position, the epidural catheter may be pulled out of the epidural space towards the skin equal to the increased distance to the epidural space in the lateral position, most likely because the catheter

may be fixed by the adhesive tape at the skin and by the thick ligamentum flavum external to the epidural space. Therefore it may be much better to tape the epidural catheter to the skin in the position in which the distance to the epidural space is greatest (lateral position) especially in obese patients [35].

5.11   Catheter Aspiration and Test Dose

The epidural catheter should be aspirated with a 2 or 5 mL empty syringe in order to detect blood and cerebrospinal fluid which are, respectively, signs of accidental intravascular and subarachnoid placement (Fig. 5.17). The aspiration test should be performed before attaching the filter to the catheter since the filter may make aspiration unreliable [36].

The aspiration of a relatively large amount of blood is an obvious sign of inadvertent epidural vein cannulation. In this case, an attempt to remove the catheter from the vein can be made by connecting the catheter to an empty 5 mL syringe and slowly withdrawing the catheter while aspirating with the syringe until the blood disappears within the catheter, indicating that the catheter has come out of the vein. Then, after having rinsed the catheter with a few millimeters of saline, the aspiration test is repeated.

It is also easy to identify a significant free flow of warm fluid from the epidural catheter as the cerebrospinal fluid.

Unfortunately a negative aspiration test cannot always rule out the inadvertent subarachnoid or intravascular positioning of an epidural catheter.

Aspiration tests may be negative due to low pressure within the epidural veins and their tendency to collapse when a negative pressure is applied, more frequently when single-lumen epidural catheters are used [37, 38]. Injection of a small amount (5 mL) of saline may dilate the collapsed vein and allows the subsequent aspiration to correctly identify the inadvertent vascular cannulation.

The aspiration of a very small amount of fluid from the epidural catheter may be due to the aspiration of a relatively large amount of saline previously injected for the loss-of-resistance technique. Techniques to distinguish between cerebrospinal fluid and saline have been described in the previous paragraph of this chapter dealing with epidural needle observation.

At least in theory, the multihole catheter can come to lie with its eyes in different anatomical spaces producing, if not recognized, combinations of intravascular, subarachnoid, and subdural injections [39].

For these reasons a test dose should follow the aspiration, to increase the chance of assessing the correct location of the epidural catheter.

The aim of the epidural test dose is to detect the inadvertent intravenous or subarachnoid placement of the epidural catheter in order to avoid, respectively, a too high or a total spinal block or local anesthetic toxicity. The test dose must be formulated to produce a rapid, reliable, and easily detected result when in one of these two situations, without compromising the safety of the mother and of the fetus.

Subarachnoid placement is relatively easy to detect. For practical reasons, the same local anesthetic that is used to produce the anesthetic block is usually chosen. Lidocaine 20–60 mg or bupivacaine (or levobupivacaine or ropivacaine) 7.5–12.5 mg is commonly used. Signs of sensory block in the lower lumbar segments and, most importantly, motor block of the legs should be sought after 3–5 min and this is considered to be specific and sensitive in almost 100% of cases. When the test dose is performed with a relatively

"high dose" of local anesthetic, such as 40–60 mg of lidocaine or 12 mg of bupivacaine, in the case of accidental intrathecal injection, a safe but complete sensory and motor block accompanied by maternal hypotension may be observed [40].

Inadvertent intravascular placement of the epidural catheter usually relies on the use of a dose of epinephrine (15 µg) capable of producing detectable changes in heart rate and blood pressure but unfortunately, in obstetrics, the intravenous injection of epinephrine has been shown to have a low positive predictive value and may be associated with side effects [41].

The ideal epidural test dose would have both high sensitivity and specificity. As sensitivity increases, more intravascular catheters would be detected. A high false-positive rate (low specificity) would lead to unnecessary manipulations or replacements of correctly positioned epidural catheters. In general, the epidural test dose has high (>90%) sensitivity but poor specificity (around 50%). Therefore, a negative test dose does not guarantee (it only decreases the probability) that the catheter is not in the intravascular or intrathecal space. Also a negative test dose does not ensure proper placement in the epidural space.

Therefore, detection of intravascular epidural catheter placement relies on repeated catheter aspiration, observation of gravity-induced fluid efflux within the catheter, failure of local anesthetic to produce the anticipated effect, and detection of early signs of toxicity by means of slow and incremental injection.

Motor response to electrical stimulation has been claimed to be a useful tool in confirming the epidural catheter location but its use has been confined to some published papers [42].

There is no single optimal way of testing epidural catheters. Direct methods, such as aspiration, should be practiced routinely. Indirect methods (local anesthetic and adrenaline) may also be considered, but can yield a false-positive result, subjecting a patient to additional unnecessary risks. No single method is 100% sensitive and there is always the possibility that catheters may migrate from the epidural space.

Even after accidental dural puncture cerebrospinal fluid may not always be aspirated.

Therefore, there is always no substitute for continued vigilance, aspirating the catheter before giving each dose, and fractionating the whole anesthetic dose in small boluses given intermittently.

5.12 Confirmation of Catheter Location in the Epidural Space

The position of the epidural catheter tip is an important factor in determining whether satisfactory epidural analgesia will be achieved, and the best confirmation of the correct positioning of an epidural catheter is the evidence of satisfactory analgesia (or anesthesia) and/or the evidence of sensory block after an adequate dose and volume of the anesthetic solution.

However, ideally, one should detect improper catheter placement at the time of epidural insertion because failure to do so adds to the duration of patient discomfort.

In addition, in spite of accurate localization of the epidural space, there is no guarantee that the catheter threaded through that needle will remain in the right place. Subsequent failure of a well-functioning epidural catheter could result from its migration out through an intervertebral foramen or from the catheter being pulled out of the epidural space, since an epidural catheter may move from its initial position with patient movement.

5.12.1 Epidural Stimulation Test

The epidural stimulation test (EST) involves electrical stimulation of nerves passing through the epidural space using a saline column in the epidural catheter.

The test is performed by connecting a nerve stimulator through an adapter to the epidural catheter connector. The epidural catheter and adapter are primed with 0.2–1 mL sterile normal saline, the negative lead of the nerve stimulator is attached to the metal hub of the adapter, and the positive lead is connected to an electrode placed over the nondependent deltoid muscle. The frequency of the nerve stimulator is set at 1 Hz with a pulse width of 200 ms. Motor or sensory response to a stimulation of 1–10 mA indicates the epidural location of the catheter tip [42]. The sensitivity of this technique, confirmed by effective epidural analgesia following local anesthetic injection, in the obstetric patient is 100% [42] while in the surgical setting it is comparable to that of the epidural pressure waveform analysis (80–100%) [43]. The epidural stimulation test (bilateral stimulation with stimulating current <1 mA) may also be useful in detecting inadvertent subarachnoid, subdural, or intravascular placement of the epidural catheter [44, 45].

However, the test may be technically difficult and cumbersome to perform in a perioperative or obstetric setting [46] and it is ineffective once local anesthetics are administered through the epidural catheter or after the patient receives neuromuscular blocking agents. Furthermore, the test cannot be relied upon in patients with preexisting neuromuscular disease. This test has not been adopted widely most likely due to these drawbacks and, in all cases, after a few promising initial studies, there are no other published reports on its routine use in obstetrics.

5.12.2 Epidural Pressure Waveform Analysis

Transducing and plotting the pressure measured in the epidural space produce a unique and reproducible waveform, which reflects heart rate and peripheral pulse waves. These waveforms are thought to originate from the spinal cord and are transmitted through the dura to the epidural space. Thus, the presence of these pulsatile waveforms in synchrony with heart rate, obtained on transducing the epidural catheter, would confirm the epidural location of the catheter. Easy availability of pressure transducers in perioperative settings could, in theory, make this an attractive method to confirm epidural location of a catheter immediately after placement or later on [47].

Fig. 5.20 Epidural pressure waveform detected by the CompuFlo Epidural Cath-Checker System: (**a**) Rhythmic pulsations indicating the correct position of the catheter into the epidural space. (**b**) Absence of rhythmic pulsations indicating the dislodgement of the catheter outside the epidural space

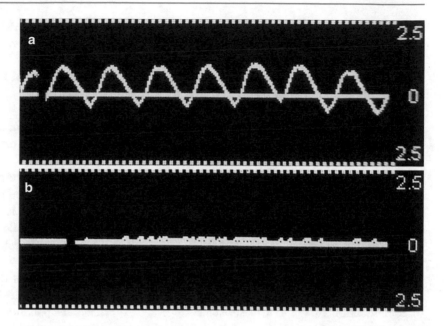

The epidural catheter is connected to a pressure transducer positioned at the midaxillary level of the patient and the test is considered positive for epidural catheter placement in the epidural space when positive pressure waveform deflections are seen on the monitor screen in synchrony with cardiac contractions (either by electrocardiogram or by pulse oximetry) after priming the epidural catheter with 5 mL saline [48].

In a preliminary report of labor epidural analgesia, the pressure waveform analysis through the epidural catheter has a sensitivity of 91%, a positive predictive value of 95%, a specificity of 83%, and a negative predictive value of 73.8% [49]. This method is not routinely and widely used, and further confirmatory studies are most welcome before its implementation in clinical practice.

Recently the CompuFlo Epidural Cath-Checker System (CCS) has been introduced.

This apparatus combines both objective pressure measurements to detect the epidural space (Sect. 6.2.2) and detection of a pulsatile pressure waveform in a single system. Utilizing a high-resolution-pressure in-line sensor the system is capable of detecting both the pressure in situ and the presence of a pulsatile waveform when present. The pulsatile waveform is representative of the detection of pressures produced by the cardiovascular system wither directly or indirectly. This in turn can be used to identify the location of a needle or a catheter within an anatomic structure such as the epidural space. This same system can also be used to determine the patency of a catheter to ensure that an obstruction or blockage of the catheter is not present. Currently, there is no other integrated device capable of determining the identification of the epidural space and the patency of a catheter. Although the preliminary data not yet published are very encouraging and promising (Fig. 5.20), this instrument, soon to be released on the market, is currently still undergoing clinical studies.

Appendix 1: Epidural Technique in Five Steps

1. Insertion of the needle

   Without moving the "landmark fingers," the epidural Tuohy needle is inserted through the skin wheal previously made exactly in the middle of the interspace.

2. Advancement of the needle

The needle must be advanced very slowly but constantly, without any interruption, in order to be able to recognize the different densities of the underlying tissues.

3. Identification of the increase of resistance (ligamentum flavum)

As soon as the point of the needle has engaged the ligamentum flavum, a feeling of a greater increase of resistance, often associated with a "crunch," is perceived. The advancement of the needle is immediately stopped.

4. Attachment of the syringe to the needle (the "self-blocking system")

Attach a disposable 10 mL loss-of-resistance syringe containing no more than 5 mL of sterile saline solution to the needle.

5. Identification of the loss of resistance (epidural space)

Exert constant, unremitting, pressure on the plunger of the syringe by the thumb of the dominant hand and advance the needle solely by means of the pressure exerted on the plunger of the syringe. As long as the needle point is in the ligamentum flavum there is a great resistance to injection and the pressure exerted by the thumb on the plunger causes the advancement of the needle. As the point of the needle emerges from the ligamentum flavum into the epidural space, the resistance suddenly disappears and the advancement of the needle immediately stops, since the driving force exerted on the piston is discharged by the sudden entry of the liquid into the epidural space

Appendix 2: Epidural Technique— The Three Immediate Safety Checks

1. Needle observation

For the appearance of spinal fluid or blood.

2. Needle aspiration

To detect cerebrospinal fluid or blood.

3. Rebound test

1–1.5 mL of air is briskly injected. The syringe must collapse

Appendix 3: Epidural Technique—Problem-Solving

Doubtful Increase in Resistance/False Loss of Resistance

1. Stop the advancement of the needle.
2. Make a slight pressure on the piston of the syringe:
   (a) If it does not determine any advancement of the piston itself and a further greater pressure on the piston causes the advancement of the needle within the tissues: the needle was correctly inserted into the ligamentum flavum.
   (b) If it causes the advancement of the piston itself and the needle does not advance under the pressure of the piston, the resistance perceived was not that of the ligamentum flavum.

In this case a false resistance may be suspected:

- Advance the needle very slowly by a few millimeters and repeat the maneuver until a resistance to moderate pressure on the piston is obtained.

Bone Contact

If:

(a) The depth at which the needle is inserted is within the range of the vertebral arch.
(b) The physician has previously perceived the typical sensation of a "crunch" due to the initial insertion of the epidural needle within the ligamentum flavum.

This means that the needle has encountered the vertebral lamina somewhere in the area where the ligamenta flava are inserted on it.

In this case:

- Redirect and advance the needle by a few millimeters (most frequently medially and cranially) until an increase of resistance is perceived.

If:

(a) The depth at which the needle is inserted is not within the range of the vertebral arch.
(b) No increase in resistance (or "crunch") has been perceived before encountering the bone:
  • Check the position of the patient.
  • Reinsert the needle with a different angle of inclination.

References

1. Dogliotti AM. Segmental peridural spinal anesthesia: a new method of block anesthesia. Am J Surg. 1933;20:107–18.
2. Walker DS, Brock-Utne JG. A comparison of simple tests to distinguish cerebrospinal fluid from saline. Can J Anaesth. 1997;44:494–7.
3. Fah A, Sutton J, Cohen V, et al. A comparison of epidural and cerebrospinal fluid glucose in parturients at term: an observational study. Int J Obstet Anesth. 2012;21:242–4.
4. Shang Y. The pH test paper: a tool for distinguish between the cerebrospinal fluid and saline. BJA. 2016;117:eLetters. https://doi.org/10.1093/bja/el_14017.
5. Tessler MJ, Wiesel S, Wahba RM, et al. A comparison of simple identification tests to distinguish cerebrospinal fluid from local anaesthetic solution. Anaesthesia. 1994;49:821–2.
6. Wantman A, Hancox N, Howell PR. Techniques for identifying the epidural space: a survey of practice among anaesthetists in the UK. Anaesthesia. 2006;61:370–5.
7. Grondin LS, Nelson K, Ross V, et al. Success of spinal and epidural labor analgesia: comparison of loss of resistance technique using air versus saline in combined spinal-epidural labor analgesia technique. Anesthesiology. 2009;111:165–72.
8. El-Behesy BA, James D, Koh KF, et al. Distinguishing cerebrospinal fluid from saline used to identify the extradural space. BJA. 1996;77:784–5.
9. Shenouda PE, Cunningham BJ. Assessing the superiority of saline versus air for use in the epidural loss of resistance technique: a literature review. Reg Anesth Pain Med. 2003;28:48–53.
10. Van de Velde M. Identification of the epidural space: stop using the loss of resistance to air technique! Acta Anaesthesiol Belg. 2006;57:51–4.
11. Murphy JD, Ouanes JP, Togioka M, et al. Comparison of air and liquid for use in loss-of-resistance technique during labor epidurals: a meta-analysis. J Anesth Clin Res. 2011;2:11. https://doi.org/10.4172/2155-6148.1000175.
12. Antibas PL, do Nascimento Junior P, Braz LG, et al. Air versus saline in the loss of resistance technique for the identification of the epidural space. Cochrane Database Syst Rev. 2014;7:CD008938. https://doi.org/10.1002/14651858.CD008938.pub2.
13. Saberski LR, Kondamuri S, Osinubi O. Identification of the epidural space: is loss of resistance to air a safe technique? A review of the complications related to the use of air. IJOA. 1997;22:3–115.
14. Todorov L, Vade Boncouer T. Etiology and use of hanging drop technique: a review. Pain Res Treat. 2014;2014:146750. https://doi.org/10.1155/2014/146750.
15. Zarzur E. Genesis of the 'true' negative pressure in the lumbar epidural space. Anaesthesia. 1984;39:1101–4.
16. Galbert MW, Marx GF. Extradural pressures in the parturient patient. Anesthesiology. 1974;40:499–502.
17. Messih MNA. Epidural space pressures during pregnancy. Anaesthesia. 1981;36:775–82.
18. Bromage PR. Epidural analgesia. Philadelphia: WB Saunders Co Pub; 1978. p. 183.
19. Blomberg RG, Jaanivald A, Walther S. Advantages of the paramedian approach for lumbar epidural analgesia with catheter technique. Anaesthesia. 1989;44:742–6.
20. Rodiera J, Calabuig R, Aliaga L, et al. Mathematical analysis of epidural space location. Int J Clin Monit Comput. 1995;12:213–7.
21. Wee MYK, Isaacs RA, Vaughan N, et al. Quantification of the pressures generated during insertion of an epidural needle in laboring women of varying body mass indices. Int J Clin Anesth Res. 2017;1:024–7.
22. Nan L, Yang XG, Lian X, et al. Full-term pregnant women have higher lumbar epidural pressure than non-pregnant women: a preliminary report. J Obstet Gynaecol. 2013;33:50–3.
23. Gibiino G, Distefano R, Camorcia M, et al. Maternal epidural pressure changes after programmed intermittent epidural bolus (PIEB) versus continuous epidural infusion (CEI). EJA. 2014;31:183–4.
24. Tran D, Hor KW, Kamani AA, et al. Instrumentation of the loss-of-resistance technique for epidural needle insertion. IEEE Trans Biomed Eng. 2009;56:820–7.
25. Beck H. The effect of the Tuohy cannula on the positioning of an epidural catheter. A radiologic analysis of the location of 175 peridural catheters. Reg Anaesth. 1990;13:42–5.
26. Igarashi T, Hirabayashi Y, Shimizu R, et al. The epidural structure changes during deep breathing. Can J Anaesth. 1999;46:850–5.
27. Mhyre JM, Greenfield ML, Tsen LC, et al. A systematic review of randomized controlled trials that evaluate strategies to avoid epidural vein cannulation during obstetric epidural catheter placement. Anesth Analg. 2009;108:1232–42.
28. Beilin Y, Bernstein HH, Zucker-Pinchoff B. The optimal distance that a multiorifice epidural catheter

should be threaded into the epidural space. Anesth Analg. 1995;81:301–3.

29. Kawaguchi T, Inoue S, Fukunaga A. Clinical analysis of failures in continuous lumbar epidural anesthesia. Masui. 1966;15:1130–6.

30. Uchino T, Miura M, Oyama Y, et al. Lateral deviation of four types of epidural catheters from the lumbar epidural space into the intervertebral foramen. J Anesth. 2016;30:583–90.

31. Afshan G, Chohan U, Khan FA, et al. Appropriate length of epidural catheter in the epidural space for postoperative analgesia: evaluation by epidurography. Anaesthesia. 2011;66:913–8.

32. Zarzur E. Displaced epidural catheter: a reason for analgesia failure. Rev Bras Anestesiol. 2002;52:251–4.

33. Clark MX, Hare K, Gorringe J, Oh T. The effect of locket epidural catheter clamp on epidural migration: a controlled trial. Anaesthesia. 2001;56:865–70.

34. Phillips DC, Macdonald R. Epidural catheter migration during labour. Anaesthesia. 1987;42:661–3.

35. Hamilton CL, Riley ET, Cohen SE. Changes in the position of epidural catheters associated with patient movement. Anesthesiology. 1997;86:778–84.

36. Charlton GA, Lawes EG. The effect of micropore filters on the aspiration test in epidural analgesia. Anaesthesia. 1991;46:573–5.

37. Kenepp NB, Gutsche BB. Inadvertent intravascular injections during lumbar epidural anesthesia. Anesthesiology. 1981;54:172–3.

38. Norris MC, Ferrenbach D, Dalman H, et al. Does epinephrine improve the diagnostic accuracy of aspiration during labor epidural analgesia? Anesth Analg. 1999;88:1073–6.

39. Collier CB, Gatt SP. A new epidural catheter. Anaesthesia. 1993;48:803–6.

40. Camorcia M. Testing the epidural catheter. Curr Opin Anaesthesiol. 2009;22:336–40.

41. Guay J. The epidural test dose: a review. Anesth Analg. 2006;102:921–9.

42. Tsui BCH, Gupta S, Finucane B. Determination of epidural catheter placement using nerve stimulation in obstetric patients. Reg Anesth. 1999;24:17–23.

43. de Medicis E, Tetrault JP, Martin R, et al. A prospective comparative study of two indirect methods for confirming the localization of an epidural catheter for postoperative analgesia. Anesth Analg. 2005;101:1830–3.

44. Tsui BC, Gupta S, Finucane B. Detection of subarachnoid and intravascular epidural catheter placement. Can J Anaesth. 1999;46:675–8.

45. Tsui BC, Gupta S, Emery D, et al. Detection of subdural placement of epidural catheter using nerve stimulation. Can J Anaesth. 2000;47:471–3.

46. Förster JG, Niemi TT, Salmenperä MT, et al. An evaluation of the epidural catheter position by epidural nerve stimulation in conjunction with continuous epidural analgesia in adult surgical patients. Anesth Analg. 2009;108:351–8.

47. Ghia J, Arora SK, Castillo M, et al. Confirmation of location of epidural catheters by epidural pressure waveform and computed tomography cathetergram. Reg Anesth Pain Med. 2001;26:337–41.

48. de Medicis E, Pelletier J, Martin R, et al. Technical report: optimal quantity of saline for epidural pressure waveform analysis. Can J Anaesth. 2007;54:818–21.

49. Al-Aami I, Derzi SH, More A, et al. Reliability of pressure waveform analysis to determine correct epidural needle placement in labouring women. Anaesthesia. 2017;72:840–4.

New Techniques and Emerging Technologies to Identify the Epidural Space

6

Over the course of the last decade, newer techniques and emerging technologies for locating and confirming entry into the epidural space have been explored to decrease failures and complications.

At the present time most of these techniques cannot be used in clinical practice since they are still experimental, not yet on the market, or not applicable in the obstetric setting. Only a few of them have been experienced in clinical studies, but their diffusion and current clinical use are unknown [1].

However, knowledge of these newer technologies is essential to guide future research in this area.

These new technologies are designed (1) to guide the needle in the epidural space through the tissues, (2) to confirm the entry of the needle into the epidural space, and (3) to confirm the epidural catheter location in the epidural space.

6.1 Guiding the Needle in the Epidural Space

Currently, the physician guides the epidural needle to the epidural space in a blind fashion, and success is dependent on the expertise of the operator. The point of needle insertion is largely identified by palpation of surface landmarks, which can be difficult in patients who are obese or who have an abnormal vertebral anatomy. The subsequent angle of insertion, speed of advancement,

degree of change in needle angle on encountering bone, etc. vary widely with the experience of the operator and the unanticipated variability in vertebral anatomy potentially leads to failure.

To overcome the blinded introduction of the needle, needle-tracking systems have been proposed and developed.

6.1.1 Ultrasound-Guided Techniques

Unlike pre-procedural scanning (Chap. 4), real-time two-dimensional (2D) ultrasonography is designed to guide the needle towards the epidural space. Unfortunately most of the experience comes exclusively from a small number of centers where it is performed by a few experienced operators. From the clinical point of view, real-time ultrasound-guided epidural insertion is technically difficult, usually requires two operators, and potentially adds the risk of introducing ultrasound gel into the epidural space.

In addition, one of its main limitations is the difficulty in visualizing the needle, or its tip, and the targeted tissue plane in the same image.

For this reason, needle-tracking navigation tools have been introduced to circumvent this limitation by improving real-time visualization of the needle.

The guidance-positioning system (Sonix GPS) [2, 3] (Fig. 6.1) uses an electromagnetic motion-

© Springer Nature Switzerland AG 2020
G. Capogna, *Epidural Technique In Obstetric Anesthesia*,
https://doi.org/10.1007/978-3-030-45332-9_6

Fig. 6.1 SonixGPS™ electromagnetic sensor arm (**a**) with SonixGPS needle with sensor filament (**b**) (from [2] with permission)

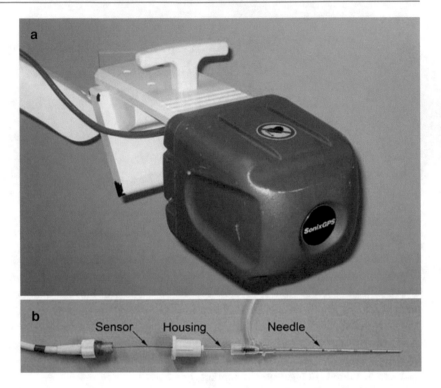

tracking system, consisting of a transmitter and one or more sensors. These sensors determine the position of the needle with respect to the ultrasound image. The position sensors located on the needle hub and the ultrasound transducer track their position with respect to the transmitter, allowing the user to have a virtual image of the needle's trajectory and the anticipated position of its tip, superimposed on the ultrasound image.

This device could be used for pre-procedural scanning as well as for real-time ultrasound-guided epidural space localization. Once the tip of the needle is at the desired point of skin entry, the GPS navigation system can be used to orient the needle such that the projected needle trajectory reaches the posterior complex. This pre-procedural scan would give information on the point of entry, direction of entry, and also the estimated depth, utilizing the on-screen calculation. Preliminary results suggest that procedural time, image quality, number of skin punctures, and number of needle redirections for successful spinal puncture are comparable with those reported with other ultrasound techniques (pre-procedural and real time) [2]. This technology requires a proprietary needle, which is currently not suitable for epidural insertion.

The high computational speed of modern machines has made it possible to obtain three-dimensional (3D) ultrasound images and to display those in real-time four-dimensional (4D) [4, 5]. As the 4D ultrasound simultaneously acquires multiple planes of view without probe repositioning, it could potentially improve the spatial orientation of the operator. A preliminary report on the cadaver [4] highlighted the challenges associated with obtaining good-quality 3D/4D ultrasound images of the spine due to the complex anatomy and strong spatially varying bony shadows and artifacts encountered. In addition, there are issues of poor resolution, reduced frame rate, and poor needle visibility with 4D images. Other important limitations are complexity and the cost involved. It is difficult to transfer the experimental cadaver experience to the clinical setting. The operator is required to concurrently interpret two ultrasound images rather than one. One single operator should hold the ultrasound probe, direct the needle, and use a reliable loss-of-resistance-to-saline technique at the same time. Current commercially available

4D ultrasound technology may offer an incremental advantage in ultrasound-guided epidural insertion by improving the spatial orientation of the operator but this comes at the price of a decreased resolution, frame rate, and needle visibility.

Due to the drawbacks of real-time 3D/4D ultrasound using current technology, investigators have tried to reconstruct the 3D vertebral anatomy of a patient. Pre-procedure off-line reconstruction can produce detailed high-resolution 3D images which can then serve as a 3D template, which can be subsequently utilized for real-time epidural space localization [6]. Pre-acquisition of these high-resolution images is however complex, expensive, and time consuming. Changes in patient position between image acquisition and procedure can alter the accuracy of the pre-acquired 3D context. Although incorporation into routine practice,

especially the obstetric one, seems very unlikely, it might have utility in patients with known difficult vertebral anatomy. Further research will evaluate its cost-effectiveness and benefit.

With advances in ultrasound technology and probe design, very small ultrasound transducers have become available and experimental (porcine) models of ultrasound through needle and needle through ultrasound have been reported.

A very-small-diameter, 40 MHz ultrasound transducer was placed in an 18-gauge Tuohy needle and used to obtain A-scan images, from the tip of the needle, from both the dura and ligamentum flavum [7]. The disappearance of the signals coming from the ligamentum flavum indicates needle entry in the epidural space (Fig. 6.2).

Alternatively, a 10 mm small-sized cylindrical ultrasound probe with a hole in the center has

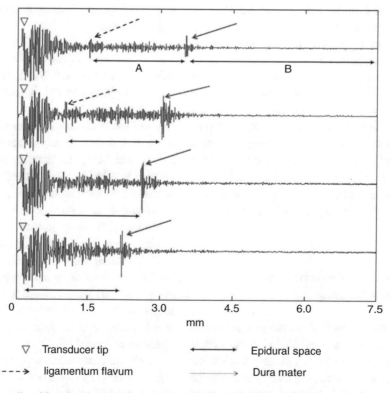

Fig. 6.2 Epidural needle with embedded high-frequency ultrasound transducer. The backscattered A-mode ultrasound signals received during the advancement of the embedded needle ultrasound transducer towards the epidural space. The top two traces show the ligamentum flavum (LF) (approximately 1.4 mm and 0.9 mm, respectively, in front of the needle transducer), and the third trace indicates that the near-field noise is overlapped with the LF signal when the LF is approximately 0.5 mm away from the needle transducer. The fourth trace indicates that the tip of the needle is about to pass through the LF and enter the epidural space. The epidural space is marked as region A. The subarachnoid space is marked as region B (from [7] with permission)

been used for the insertion of the epidural needle and the specific lumbar interspaces were accurately identified [8].

Both these techniques have the advantage of providing real-time guidance and can be performed by a single operator, but they need special specific equipment. Though promising, the absence of any human studies makes the future of this technology uncertain.

6.1.2 Augmented Reality System for Epidural Anesthesia

A prototype of an augmented reality system has been developed to help the identification of the lumbar vertebral levels (augmented reality system for epidural anesthesia, AREA) [9]. The system consists of an ultrasound transducer tracked in real time by a trinocular camera system, an automatic ultrasound panorama generation module that provides an extended view of the lumbar vertebrae, an image-processing technique that automatically identifies the vertebral levels in the panorama image, and a graphical interface that overlays the identified levels on a live camera view of the patient's back. This prototype has been validated by a comparison with standard ultrasound in volunteers but it has never been used in clinical practice. In addition, the ability of these systems to identify structures in the presence of uncommon or distorted anatomy is unknown.

6.1.3 Acoustic Radiation Force Impulse Imaging

An important drawback of ultrasounds is the difficulty in obtaining a clear image of the needle and clear differentiation of the nerves from the surrounding soft tissues, which have similar acoustic impedances. Acoustic radiation force imaging (ARFI) differentiates tissues based on their elasticity, unlike traditional ultrasonography which differentiates tissue based on acoustic impedances [10] (Fig. 6.3). ARFI image contrast is derived from differences in the mechani-

cal properties of tissue, rather than the acoustic properties. ARFI images are generated using a diagnostic ultrasound system and therefore co-registered B-mode and ARFI images are acquired concurrently. The needle visualization in ARFI images is independent of the needle-insertion angle and also extends needle visibility out of plane.

While ARFI images provide enhanced needle contrast due to the much larger stiffness and fixed nature of the needle as compared to the surrounding tissue, they do not show the same vascular and nerve landmarks that clinicians look for when performing regional anesthesia. Combining the improved needle contrast from ARFI imaging and surrounding tissue information from B-mode could aid visualization within the complex vertebral sonoanatomy [11]. Unfortunately this technology requires considerable research and development before it could be available commercially.

6.2 Identifying the Entry into the Epidural Space

None of the automated epidural devices described in Chap. 4 have currently replaced the traditional loss-of-resistance technique. However, in the attempt to eliminate the subjective nature of loss of resistance, novel markers to identify entry into the epidural space have been introduced.

Some [12] have proposed connecting the Tuohy needle to a regular intravenous set (IV) with a normal saline bag and pressurizing the fluid bag to 50 mmHg using a pressure bag. The entry into the epidural space would be determined by resulting in flow of fluid into the epidural space, seen as fluid dripping in the fluid chamber of the IV set.

A similar, but more sophisticated, system is the acoustic puncture assist device (APAD) [13] which quantifies the pressure at the epidural needle tip and provides real-time auditory and visual displays of the pressure waveforms, during epidural space localization. Once the needle tip is advanced through the skin, the APAD is connected to the needle hub, which maintains

Fig. 6.3 Acoustic radiation force impulse (ARFI) imaging-based needle visualization. B-mode images of an angled 18G needle in a 200-bloom graphite phantom at different angles with respect to the horizontal without (top row) and with (bottom row) needle visualization algorithm applied. Column 1 [(**a**) and (**d**)] shows a 10° angle above the horizontal, column 2 [(**b**) and (**e**)] shows a 16° angle, and column 3 [(**c**) and (**f**)] shows a 32° angle. The green X in each image of the bottom row shows the location of the needle tip as determined by bisecting the phantom in the needle-imaging plane (from [11] with permission)

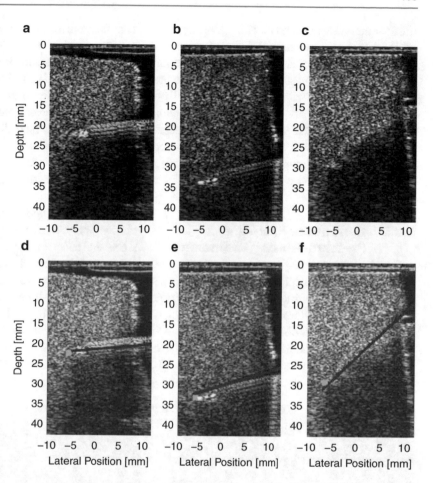

a pressurized fluid column through the epidural needle. As the epidural needle is advanced, the pressure from the column is measured and transmitted as auditory signals and visually displayed as pressure tracings. Entry into the epidural space results in a sudden drop in pressure on the visual display as well as a distinct fall in the tone of the audio output. The lack of demonstrable superiority to the traditional loss-of-resistance technique has limited the use of such a device in routine clinical practice.

6.2.1   Epidural Pressure Checker

The concept underlying the design of this device is that a specific area of the human body exists as a vacuum with no pressure shift such that the digital sensor recognizes the pressure shift between the ligamentum flavum and the epidural space.

The epidural pressure checker (Epi-Detection®) is designed to detect the epidural space by perceiving the pressure shift to a negative value [14].

This device is composed of a printed circuit board (PCB) containing a micro-electromechanical system (MEM) pressure sensor and polycarbonate spouting that connects to a Tuohy needle. The epidural pressure checker perceives the negative pressure with a preset pressure threshold and alarms with sound and light. The pressure changes are displayed by the LED as green (ready) and blue (detection) (Fig. 6.4) so that the operator can identify the puncture needle in order to reach the exact position of the epidural space. When a Tuohy needle connected to the epidural pressure checker penetrates the ligamentum flavum and encounters the epidural space, the negative pressure of the epidural space is transferred to the epidural pressure checker via the inner cannula of the needle. The allowable error of the device ranges from −0.5 to +0.5 mbar.

One possible limitation is that the epidural pressure checker might not detect a pressure change in patients with a weak or absent ligamentum flavum, or above or below its detection range, and in this case it can result in false negatives or false positives. The device has been used in non-obstetric patients and further clinical trials are currently underway.

6.2.2 Continuous Real-Time Pressure-Sensing Technology

The CompuFlo® Epidural Instrument is a computer-controlled drug delivery system capable of distinguishing different tissue types by providing continuously real-time "exit-pressure" data at the needle tip and that has been validated as a useful tool in detecting the epidural space [15–17].

This instrument uses the continuous real-time pressure-sensing technology, an algorithm to determine the pressure at the tip of the needle via a continuous fluid path. The pressure is a feedback loop and controller to the system, thus regulating the electromechanical motor which controls the flow rate and the fluid dispensed by the system. An audible feedback and a visual graphic of exit pressure are provided to the healthcare practitioner enabling the operator to focus on the injection site (Fig. 6.5).

This way the physician has an objective, quantitative method to identify the epidural space since the entry of the needle into the epidural space may be seen through the graphic display which shows a typical and reliable pattern, and, at the same time, it may also be confirmed by the clear changes of the audible tone.

Using the CompuFlo® the entry of the needle into the ligamentum flavum is indicated by a great increase in pressure on the visual display with a

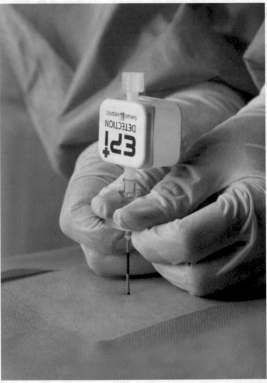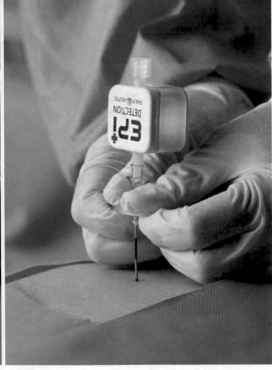

Fig. 6.4 The epidural pressure checker (Epi-Detection®). The pressure changes are displayed by the LED as green (ready) and blue (detection)

Fig. 6.5 Continuous real-time pressure-sensing technology: the CompuFlo® epidural instrument

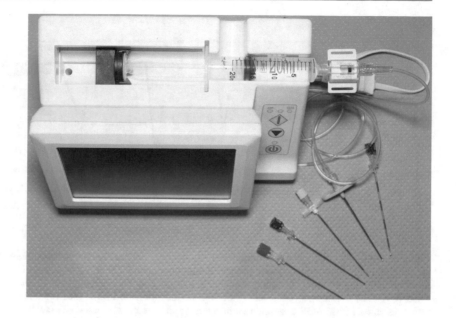

Pressure - Volume

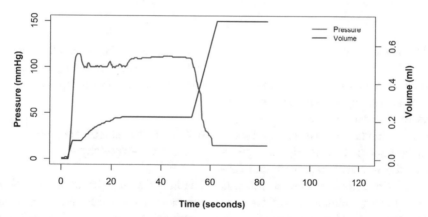

Fig. 6.6 Typical pressure and volume display observed on the CompuFlo® epidural computer-controlled anesthesia system during epidural space identification. The entry of the needle into the ligamentum flavum is indicated by a great increase in pressure, while a sudden drop in pressure followed by formation of a low-pressure plateau indicates that the epidural space has been reached. Injection of saline halts when the preset pressure limit (130 mmHg) is reached

simultaneous increase of the pitch of the audible tone, while the entry of the needle into the epidural space results in a brisk drop in pressure and a distinct fall in the tone of the audio output. A drop in pressure sustained for more than 5 s is deemed to be consistent with entry into the epidural space. Typical curves can be obtained (Fig. 6.6).

CompuFlo® may also help the physician to differentiate the false loss of resistance due to the location of the epidural needle within the epidural region tissues and the true loss of resistance due to the penetration of the needle in the epidural space with a sensitivity of 0.83 and a specificity of 0.81 [18] (Fig. 6.7).

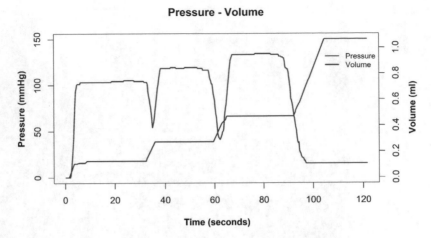

Fig. 6.7 Typical pressure and volume display observed on the CompuFlo® epidural computer-controlled anesthesia system during epidural space identification showing false losses of resistance (false LOR) during needle advancement. A false LOR is defined as an increase of pressure followed by a small drop in pressure (typically less than 50% of the maximum pressure) that is either not sustained or inconclusive of representing a "low and stable pressure plateau." If the pressure rapidly increased after a drop of pressure this is identified as a false loss of resistance and the operator elects to continue to advance the epidural needle

6.2.3   Bioimpedance

Bioimpedance is a measure of the opposition to the flow of alternating current. This property can be used to differentiate several tissue types including muscle and fat [19]. The epidural space has a higher fat content than its adjoining structures such as the ligamentum flavum and subarachnoid or intrathecal compartments, aiding in its identification using bioimpedance. Change in bioimpedance measured with an epidural needle may identify the epidural space and the ligamentum flavum. The bioimpedance measurement just prior to loss of resistance is assumed to be the ligamentum flavum. While there is variation in absolute values between patients, the delta in value between the ligamentum flavum and the epidural space is quite stable [20]. Bioimpedance has been used in association with loss of resistance and confirmed with fluoroscopic dye; therefore its role as a sole method for localization needs to be further investigated. At present it could serve, in theory, as a complementary tool during epidural localization when the position of the needle tip is in question. The potential advantages of this technique are that it can be performed by a single operator and requires inexpensive equipment.

6.2.4   Optical Reflectance Spectroscopy

The intensity of light reflected or absorbed by a particular tissue varies and depends on the tissue composition. Optical reflectance spectroscopy (ORS) uses this property to differentiate various tissues based on their optical absorption. The optical spectra may be measured at the needle tip using a specialized stylet introduced through the epidural needle [21] or by using used optical fibers embedded within the needle [22]. Optical spectra are significantly different between epidural space and ligamentum flavum (Fig. 6.8) and thus could serve as a tool to identify the epidural location of the needle tip. Epidural placements in porcine models have 95% success confirmed by epidurography but these results were obtained by operators with sufficient expertise in interpreting ORS [23].

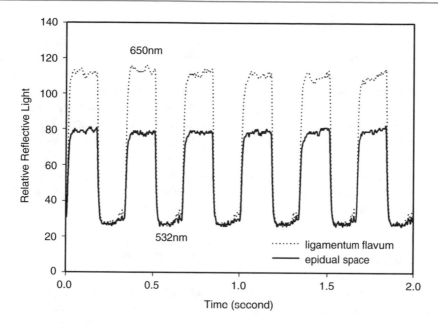

Fig. 6.8 Fiber-optic-guided insertion using two wavelengths. The reflective signals at 650 and 532 nm are shown while the stylet reaches the ligamentum flavum and epidural space. The *y*-axis is the magnitude of light reflected from the tissues (the peaks represent the 650 nm wavelength whereas the troughs indicate the 532 nm wavelength). The *x*-axis indicates the time course of the modulation for 650 and 532 nm during the insertion of the needle into the tissue. (*Dotted line*) The reflected light when the needle is located in the ligamentum flavum and (*solid line*) the light reflected from the epidural space. The two lines illustrate the reflectance that is obtained at different times (i.e., when the needle is in two different locations) but are superimposed to provide a visual comparison (from [23] with permission)

Although it appears to be a promising technique, it has not yet been tried in humans.

6.2.5 Optical Coherence Tomography

Optical coherence tomography (OCT) is the optical analogue of B-mode ultrasonography, but measures time delay and magnitude of light, instead of sound. The light reflected back from tissue is used to determine the depth of penetration and then to create 2D and 3D images of the imaged tissue. Though the depth of imaging is limited to approximately 2 mm, it is adequate for the identification of structures immediately at the tip of the needle [24].

This technique has been used in animal studies to prevent inadvertent intraneural injection while performing transforaminal nerve root injections [25] but its use in epidural space localization has only been speculated and never been explored.

6.3 Confirming the Catheter Location in Epidural Space

In spite of the accurate localization of the epidural space, there is no guarantee that the catheter threaded through that needle would remain in it. Failure could result from migration of the epidural catheter out through an intervertebral foramen or from the catheter being pulled out of the epidural space.

The position of the epidural catheter tip is an important factor in determining whether satisfactory epidural analgesia will be achieved. New techniques for identifying the location of the epidural catheter tip during epidural placement or subsequently to investigate the secondary failure have been proposed.

6.3.1   Near-Infrared Tracking System

The near-infrared tracking system consists of a fiber-optic wire, placed in an epidural catheter, which emits an infrared signal allowing its visualization with an infrared camera. It has been successfully used in cadavers to facilitate the threading of an epidural catheter to a desired vertebral level; however, the signal decreases in obese patients, and when the catheter passes under lamina or diverges from the midline. Its role in confirming the epidural position of a catheter is uncertain [26].

6.3.2   Ultrasound

Ultrasonography has been used to accurately locate the epidural catheter position within the epidural space in infants, by identifying the movement of dura, from expansion of epidural space during local anesthetic injection through the epidural catheter [27].

The use of these methods has not been reported in adults or in obstetric patients, but would likely be hampered by poor image quality from ossified vertebrae.

6.3.3   Optical Fiber Technology for Epidural Needle (OFTEN)

This system is based on a customized optical fiber sensor, the so-called fiber Bragg grating (FBG). FBG detects in real time the density of the tissues encountered by the needle during its advancement. FBG is integrated inside a conventional epidural catheter which is, in turn, inserted into the epidural needle. Through real-time measurements, the fiber Bragg grating integrated inside the needle lumen is able to effectively perceive the typical force drop occurring when the needle enters the epidural space.

Animal tests hypothesize that this device could be able to assist clinicians not only in the performance of the epidural block, but also in the assessment of the correct positioning of the epidural catheter into the epidural space by monitoring the intensity of the FBG back-reflected signal [28] (Fig. 6.9).

6.4   Conclusion

None of the newer techniques have currently replaced the traditional loss-of-resistance technique. Pre-procedural ultrasound is increasingly being used as a routine or rescue method when a patient with difficult anatomy is encountered. Among the new techniques, continuous real-time pressure-sensing technology is the only one that has been successfully validated and used in an adequate number of patients and that therefore may be considered as a new, promising tool.

Several of the newer technologies need further characterization of safety profile and proof of a favorable cost-benefit profile. Demonstration of a lower complication rate would require larger studies, especially since the traditional technique itself is associated with a low complication rate. The majority of the newer technologies are in the early stages of development and, at the present time, it is difficult to have an accurate insight into their potential.

Fig. 6.9 Optical fiber technology for epidural needle (OFTEN). (**a**) The device. (**b**) Signal recorded during the needle placement. (**c**) Signal recorded in case of kinking of the catheter (courtesy of Dr. A. Ricciardi)

a

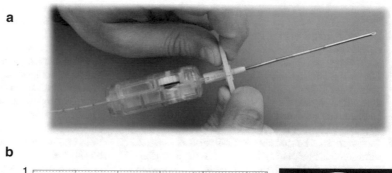

b

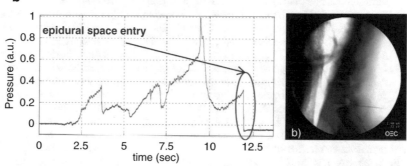

c

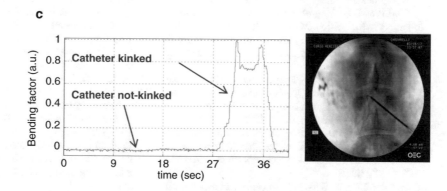

References

1. Grau T, Leipold RW, Fatehi S, et al. Real-rime ultrasonic observation of combined spinal–epidural anesthesia. Eur J Anaesthesiol. 2004;21:25–3.

2. Brinkmann S, Tang R, Sawka A, et al. Single-operator real-time ultrasound-guided spinal injection using Sonix GPSTM: a case series. Can J Anaesth. 2013;60:896–901.

3. Wong SW, Niazi AU, Chin KJ, et al. Real-time ultrasound- guided spinal anesthesia using the SonixGPS®

needle tracking system: a case report. Can J Anaesth. 2013;60:50–3.

4. Belavy D, Ruitenberg MJ, Brijball RB. Feasibility study of real-time three-/four-dimensional ultrasound for epidural catheter insertion. Br J Anaesth. 2011;107:438–45.

5. Clendenen SR, Robards CB, Clendenen NJ, et al. Real-time 3-dimensional ultrasound-assisted infraclavicular brachial plexus catheter placement: Implications of a new technology. Anesthesiol Res Pract. 2010;2010. pii: 208025.

6. Rafii-Tari H, Abolmaesumi P, Rohling R. Panorama ultrasound for guiding epidural anesthesia: a feasibility study. In: Taylor RH, Yang GZ, editors. Information processing in computer assisted interventions LNCS 6689. Berlin: Springer Science and Business Media; 2011. p. 179–89.

7. Chiang HK, Zhou Q, Mandell MS, et al. Eyes in the needle: novel epidural needle with embedded high-frequency ultrasound transducer—epidural access in porcine model. Anesthesiology. 2011;114:1320–4.

8. Chen GS, Chang YC, Chang Y, et al. A prototype axial ultrasound needle guide to reduce epidural bone contact. Anaesthesia. 2014;69:746–51.

9. Ashab HA, Lessoway VA, Khallaghi S, et al. AREA: an augmented reality system for epidural anaesthesia. Conf Proc IEEE Eng Med Biol Soc. 2012;26:59–63.

10. Palmeri ML, Dahl JJ, MacLeod DB, et al. On the feasibility of imaging peripheral nerves using acoustic radiation force impulse imaging. Ultrason Imaging. 2009;31:172–82.

11. Rotemberg V, Palmeri M, Rosenzweig S, et al. Acoustic radiation force impulse (ARFI) imaging-based needle visualization. Ultrason Imaging. 2011;33:1–16.

12. Samhan YM, El-Sabae HH, Khafagy HF, et al. A pilot study to compare epidural identification and catheterization using a saline-filled syringe versus a continuous hydrostatic pressure system. J Anesth. 2013;27:607–10.

13. Lechner TJ, van Wijk MG, Maas AJ, et al. Clinical results with the acoustic puncture assist device, a new acoustic device to identify the epidural space. Anesth Analg. 2003;96:1183–7.

14. Lee N, Park SS, Yeul G, et al. Utility of an epidural pressure checker in the administration of translaminar epidural blocks. Asian J Pain. 2016;2:6–9.

15. Ghelber O, Gebhard RE, Vora S, et al. Identification of the epidural space using pressure measurement with the CompuFlo injection pump—a pilot study. Reg Anesth Pain Med. 2008;33:346–52.

16. Capogna G, Camorcia M, Coccoluto A, et al. Experimental validation of the CompuFlo epidural controlled system to identify the epidural space and its clinical use in difficult obstetric cases. Int J Obstet Anesth. 2018;36:28–33.

17. Gebhard RE, Moelter-Bertram T, Dobeki D, et al. Objective epidural space identification using continuous real-time pressure sensing technology: a randomized controlled comparison with fluoroscopy and traditional loss of resistance. Anesth Analg. 2019;129:1319–27. https://doi.org/10.1213/ANE.0000000000003873.

18. Vaira P, Camorcia M, Palladino T, et al. Differentiating false loss of resistance from true loss of resistance while performing the epidural block with the CompuFlo® epidural instrument. Anesthesiol Res Pract. 2019;3:518590. https://doi.org/10.1155/2019/5185901.

19. Kalvøy H, Frich L, Grimnes S, et al. Impedance-based tissue discrimination for needle guidance. Physiol Meas. 2009;30:129–40.

20. Patteson SK, Ollis J, Lehmann L, et al. Bioimpedance for identification of the epidural space. Anesthesiology. 2011;A1261.

21. Ting CK, Chang Y. Technique of fiber optics used to localize epidural space in piglets. Opt Express. 2010;18:11138–47.

22. Desjardins AE, Hendriks BH, van der Voort M, et al. Epidural needle with embedded optical fibers for spectroscopic differentiation of tissue: ex vivo feasibility study. Biomed Opt Express. 2011;2:1452–61.

23. Ting CK, Tsou MY, Chen PT, et al. A new technique to assist epidural needle placement: fiberoptic-guided insertion using two wavelengths. Anesthesiology. 2010;112:1128–35.

24. Zysk AM, Nguyen FT, Oldenburg AL, et al. Optical coherence tomography: a review of clinical development from bench to bedside. J Biomed Opt. 2007;12:051403.

25. Raphael DT, Yang C, Tresser N, et al. Images of spinal nerves and adjacent structures with optical coherence tomography: preliminary animal studies. J Pain. 2007;8:767–73.

26. Chiu SC, Bristow SJ, Gofeld M. Near-infrared tracking system for epidural catheter placement: a feasibility study. Reg Anesth Pain Med. 2012;37:354–6.

27. Willschke H, Marhofer P, Bösenberg A, et al. Epidural catheter placement in children: comparing a novel approach using ultrasound guidance and a standard loss-of-resistance technique. Br J Anaesth. 2006;97:200–7.

28. Carotenuto B, Ricciardi A, Micco A, et al. Optical fiber technology enables smart needles for epidurals: an in-vivo swine study. Biomed Opt Express. 2019;10:1351–64.

Combined Spinal-Epidural Technique

The combined spinal-epidural block (CSE) has the potential ability to combine the rapidity, density, and reliability of the subarachnoid block with the flexibility of the continuous epidural block to titrate a desired sensory level, vary the intensity of the block, control the duration of anesthesia, and deliver postoperative analgesia.

7.1 History

"By combining the two methods many of the disadvantages of both methods are eliminated and their advantages are enhanced to an almost incredible degree." With these words Angelo Luigi Soresi (1877–1951) described in 1937 his "epi-subdural technique" [1], obtained by first injecting a dose of local anesthetic epidurally and, after advancing the needle inside the subarachnoid space, injecting the spinal dose. "Epi-subdural anesthesia" did not involve the placement of an epidural catheter, and Soresi concluded his paper stating that "the hanging drop method renders epi-subdural anesthesia the safest procedure giving perfect surgical anesthesia, ideal relaxation, and eliminating practically all postoperative pain and distress."

Forty years later, Ioan Curelaru was the first to publish a study on CSE anesthesia in 1979 [2]. In his study CSE anesthesia was performed in two different interspaces: first, the epidural catheter was placed and then a subarachnoid injection was carried out two levels below the level of the epidural catheter insertion. Curelaru discussed in his paper that CSE anesthesia confers several advantages, including high-quality conduction anesthesia that could be extended as needed, prolonged postoperative analgesia, analgesia covering a satisfactory number of dermatomes, minimal local anesthetic toxicity, and absence of pulmonary complications. In addition, he also discussed the drawbacks of the technique, including the need for two lumbar punctures, prolonged procedural time for the double procedure, and difficulty locating the subarachnoid space after inserting a catheter in the epidural space.

A few years later, Brownridge, from Australia, in 1981 [3] in order to increase intraoperative maternal comfort, proposed using a combination of epidural and subarachnoid block for elective cesarean section by introducing an epidural catheter in the lateral position and, after having given a test dose, performing a subarachnoid block at a lower lumbar level with a 26-gauge spinal needle.

In 1982 Coates, from the UK [4], first reported a technical innovation that he called "single-space technique" by inserting a spinal needle through the epidural needle and injecting the local anesthetic in the subarachnoid space first, and then placing an epidural catheter, in this way

© Springer Nature Switzerland AG 2020
G. Capogna, *Epidural Technique In Obstetric Anesthesia*,
https://doi.org/10.1007/978-3-030-45332-9_7

introducing the so-called needle-through-needle technique.

In 1986, Rawal, in Sweden [5], described the "sequential CSE technique" for cesarean delivery. With this technique, after the spinal block was "fixed" (about 15 min) and the extent of analgesia noted, the block was extended to the T4 dermatome by injecting fractionated doses of bupivacaine in the epidural catheter.

CSE for labor analgesia was first introduced in the early 1990s by Barbara Morgan in London [6].

Since then, over the years, a variety of specialized combined spinal-epidural needles have been devised and a number of techniques described to refine this procedure.

7.2   Classification

There may be a number of different approaches, differently classified according to the type of the needle and the approach used (Fig. 7.1). The possible approaches are basically two: the single-interspace technique, if the epidural and the spinal punctures are performed in the same interspace, usually with a single needle (needle-through-needle) or, very rarely, with two different needles, and the double-interspace technique when the epidural and spinal punctures are accomplished by using two separate interspaces, with two different needles.

Performing both the epidural and spinal injection at the same interspace with the needle-

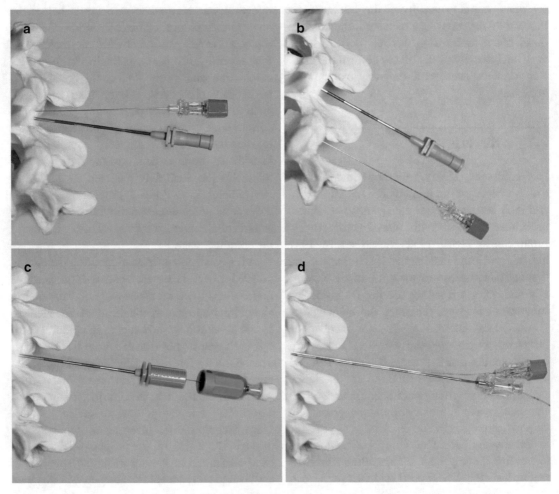

Fig. 7.1 CSE: possible approaches. (**a**) Single-interspace technique with two different needles. (**b**) Double-interspace technique (two separate interspaces, with two different needles). (**c**) Single-interspace technique with a single needle (needle-through-needle). (**d**) Single-interspace technique with a single needle (needle-beside-needle)

through-needle technique requires infiltration with local anesthetic only once. When using this technique, the epidural needle is placed first, to serve as introducer for the spinal needle at the same interspace. Then, after the epidural catheter is advanced, the spinal needle is advanced in order to puncture the dura and allow the subarachnoid injection. With this technique, epidural catheter damage caused with the spinal needle during dural puncture is a theoretical possible complication.

The technique using two different interspaces requires two local anesthetic infiltrations, and does not require specialized, more expensive needles, but confers the advantage that it allows the use of an epidural test dose to confirm the appropriate placement of the epidural catheter before the spinal injection and avoids potential puncture of the epidural catheter by the spinal needle.

However, despite these presumed advantages, there is no robust evidence in favor of one of them.

7.3 Single-Interspace Technique

7.3.1 Two Needles in the Same Interspace

In theory, the epidural as well as the spinal needles may be separately placed in the same interspace to perform the epidural puncture first and subarachnoid puncture thereafter or vice versa, offering the physician different choices of positioning the epidural catheter and performing the spinal block (Fig. 7.1). This technique is however rarely performed.

7.3.2 Needle-Through-Needle (Single Channel)

This is the most commonly used technique. After the epidural space is identified using an epidural needle, the epidural needle serves as introducer, and a fine spinal needle is advanced through the epidural needle, beyond its tip, until it punctures the dura (Fig. 7.2). Medications are first injected in the subarachnoid space, and then the epidural catheter is inserted.

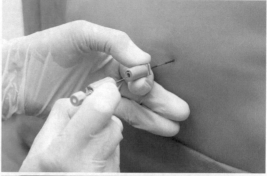
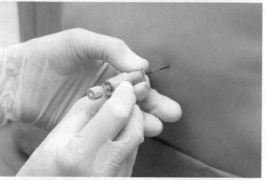
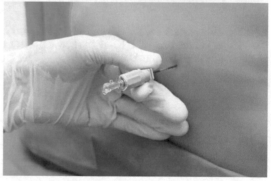

Fig. 7.2 Single-interspace technique with a single needle (needle-through-needle). After the epidural space is identified using an epidural needle, the epidural needle serves as the introducer, and a fine spinal needle is advanced through the epidural needle, beyond its tip, until it punctures the dura

Although it is possible to combine a plain Tuohy needle with a longer, thinner spinal needle to perform the procedure, special commercial "all-in-one" kits have become available. Lockable CSE sets provide safe and stable conditions and a good success rate of subarachnoid block [7] (Fig. 7.3). CSEcure® locking needle sets enable the spinal and epidural needle relationship to be stabilized during injection of the spinal anesthetic to prevent

Fig. 7.3 Lockable CSE sets. They provide safe and stable conditions and a good success rate of subarachnoid block

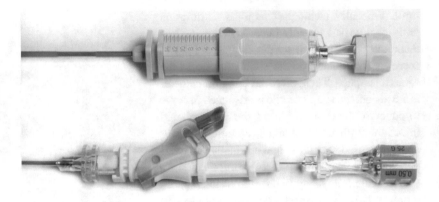

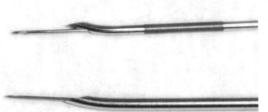

Fig. 7.4 An epidural needle with an additional aperture ("back eye") in the heel of its bevel, to allow the sleeved spinal needle to pass through

movement of the spinal needle. A scale indicates spinal needle extension beyond the epidural needle tip. Once the hubs are locked, the spinal needle is free to rotate 360°, providing the physician with the flexibility to inject spinal medication in any direction. The clear spinal needle hub provides easy and rapid identification of CSF flashback, helping to confirm correct needle placement.

With the needle-through-needle technique, there is a theoretical concern about the tip of the spinal needle scraping the bevel of the Tuohy needle and the inner wall of the epidural needle and thereby leading to deposition of metal particles in the epidural and/or subarachnoid spaces with possible subsequent neurological sequelae [8]. Even if there is no evidence of additional metal particles produced by the needle-through-needle technique [9], in order to avoid this theoretical risk, new types of needles have been introduced (Hanaoka needles) (Fig. 7.4).

The Espocan® combined spinal epidural needle is an epidural needle with an additional

aperture ("back eye") in the heel of its bevel, to allow the sleeved spinal needle to pass through. The spinal needle is introduced through the proximal port of the epidural needle to exit at the "back eye" and after dural puncture and drug administration the spinal needle is withdrawn, and the catheter inserted. The larger diameter of the catheter causes it to pass through the usual bevel opening. To accomplish proper passage through the "back eye," however, the distal end of the spinal needle must face the same way as the bevel opening of the epidural needle. To facilitate this proper passage a plastic sleeve for the spinal needle has been introduced by the Espocan® system, where the plastic sleeve keeps the spinal needle centrally in the epidural needle and guides it through the back eye. As the spinal needle is advanced through the Tuohy needle its centering sleeve aligns the spinal needle with the back-eye lumen to help prevent an over-the-curve placement. The epidural catheter is eventually directed through the Tuohy curve, away from the dura puncture site to lessen the chance of intrathecal catheter placement.

Lockable CSE sets are commercially available also with "back-eye" needles (Fig. 7.3).

7.3.3 Needle-Beside-Needle (Double Channel)

To avoid friction between the spinal and the epidural needles and to ensure that dural puncture is separated from epidural catheter placement double-barrel, parallel epidural-spinal needles have been designed (Fig. 7.1).

The first to be introduced onto the market in the 1990s were the Eldor needle (an epidural needle with a spinal conduit alongside) [10] (Fig. 7.5) and the Coombs epidural-spinal needle (a multilumen construction) [11].

Both are specialized needles for combined spinal-epidural anesthesia. The epidural catheter can be inserted before the spinal anesthetic injection. Their use avoids the theoretical risks of the needle-through-needle technique such as the danger of epidural catheter protrusion through the dural hole made by the spinal needle and metallic microparticle production while the spinal needle passes through the bent epidural needle tip. First, the spinal needle is introduced into the guide needle as far as the distal end of the latter. Then, the epidural specialized needle is introduced into the selected intervertebral space and the epidural space is located using the well-known indicator methods. After that the epidural catheter is introduced into the epidural space, confirming its position by the test dose technique. Then, the spinal needle is slowly pushed in to puncture the dura and cerebrospinal fluid is obtained. The anesthetic solution is injected through the spinal needle into the subarachnoid space. Subsequently, the spinal needle is slowly withdrawn from the guide needle, and the epidural specialized needle is withdrawn, leaving the epidural catheter in position in the epidural space.

Other specialized needles have been introduced over time, such as the Rusch Epistar CSE needle®, which is a Tuohy needle with a shape that prevents the catheter from being damaged by the spinal needle and assures stable insertion of both components [12].

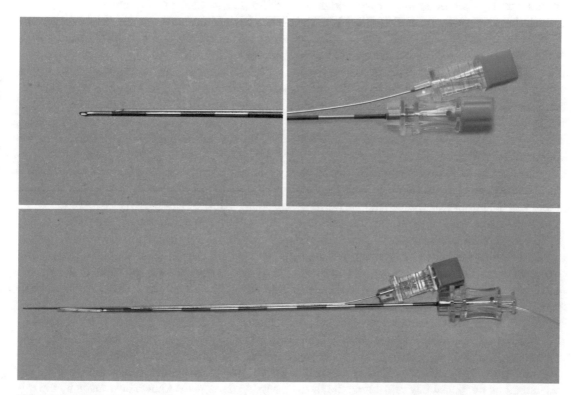

Fig. 7.5 Double-barrel, parallel epidural-spinal needle (Eldor needle). First, the spinal needle is introduced into the guide needle. Then, the epidural needle is introduced into the selected intervertebral space and the epidural space is located. After that, the epidural catheter is introduced into the epidural space, confirming its position by the test dose technique. Then, the spinal needle is slowly pushed in to puncture the dura, cerebrospinal fluid is obtained, and the spinal anesthetic solution is injected

These kinds of specialized needles may be however uncomfortably large, and have not gained widespread popularity.

7.4 Double-Interspace Technique

In this technique, the two components of CSE (spinal and epidural injection) are performed using two separate needles, at different intervertebral spaces (Fig. 7.1). This allows the epidural catheter to be placed and tested before subarachnoid block is initiated, which is not possible with needle-through-needle CSE. However, there is a theoretical risk that the spinal needle may strike the epidural catheter during placement, damaging the needle or the catheter. To prevent this unlikely complication, an alternative, but slightly complicated, technique has been proposed: a spinal needle is placed as low as possible in the selected interspace and the CSF identified. The spinal needle stylet is replaced, and an epidural needle is placed cephalad and the epidural catheter is then placed. The spinal needle stylet is removed and subarachnoid blockade performed. The technique allows placement of the epidural catheter before subarachnoid injection but does not require placing the spinal needle with an epidural catheter in situ [13].

The double-interspace technique may allow an epidural catheter placement in both the thoracic and the lumbar area, depending on the location of the pain, while the subarachnoid injection is still done in the lumbar area.

By using two different interspaces, one in the epidural space and one in the subarachnoid space, also two catheters may be positioned on the same patient. Having both an epidural and a subarachnoid catheter confers certain advantages, in that both spinal anesthesia and epidural analgesia can be extended or prolonged, as needed for surgery and postoperative analgesia. Another potential advantage is the possibility of titrating the intrathecal dose of the local anesthetic to the desired dermatomal level and testing the correct position of the epidural catheter before injecting the drugs. However, due to concerns about the severe risk of inadvertent epidural injection of local anesthetic through the subarachnoid, rather than through the epidural catheter, the dual-catheter technique is rarely used [14, 15].

7.5 Optimal Length of the Spinal Needle Beyond the Epidural Needle Tip

The distance from the tip of the epidural needle to the posterior wall of the dural sac in the midline varies considerably among patients (0.3–1.03 cm) [16, 17].

In addition, the anteroposterior diameter of the dural sac varies considerably during flexion and extension of the spinal column. For example, at the L3–L4 level, the diameter increases from a range of 9–20 mm in extension to a range of 11–25 mm in flexion [18]. Therefore, a minimum of 13–15 mm length of the spinal needle protrusion beyond the epidural needle tip is recommended for the CSE sets for a reasonably high success rate [19, 20].

Also, because of the needle design, the length of protrusion for needles with side orifice should be greater than that for end-orifice needles [21]. However, these considerations are only valid when the epidural puncture is performed in the midline.

7.6 Risk of Epidural Catheter Subarachnoid Migration

The risk of the epidural catheter penetrating the dura mater through the hole made by the spinal needle could be a major concern with CSE. Separate-needle CSE where the epidural catheter is placed first or distant from dural puncture can avoid this problem but needle-through-needle CSE cannot. An epidural catheter may enter the subarachnoid space during CSE by passing through the known hole made by the spinal needle or through an unrecognized hole made by the epidural needle. Rotation of the Tuohy needle after spinal placement to redirect the epidural catheter away from the dural hole may increase the ease of dural puncture and, therefore, is not advisable [22].

However, a cadaveric study demonstrated that it was impossible to force an 18-gauge epidural catheter through the dural hole after a single dural puncture made by a 25-gauge spinal needle. After multiple dural punctures with the spinal needle, the epidural catheter penetrates the perforated dura in 5% of cases. The epidural catheter penetrates the dural hole made by the Tuohy needle in 45% of cases [23].

Subarachnoid catheter passage is unlikely in the presence of intact dura or after an uncomplicated combined spinal epidural with a 25-gauge Whitacre needle. Rather, unintentional subarachnoid catheter passage suggests the presence of dural damage with the epidural needle [24].

7.7   Subarachnoid Spread of Epidurally Administered Drugs and the Dural Puncture Technique (DPE)

Occasionally extensive block and hypotension may occur after inadvertent dural puncture and the subsequent epidural injection of local anesthetics and the subarachnoid spread of solution from the epidural space may be confirmed radiologically [25].

A bolus solution of drug injected via the epidural catheter has the potential to leak through the dural puncture into the subarachnoid space, but this has been demonstrated only for relatively large-bore needles, and, in addition, this is not usually a clinically significant problem [26–28].

The possible passage of epidural medications through a dural puncture is the basis of the dural puncture epidural (DPE) technique: after performing CSE via the needle-through-needle technique, the spinal needle is withdrawn without any subarachnoid drug administration. Then, an epidural catheter is placed to administer analgesic solutions through it. However, whether this method may improve the quality of epidural labor analgesia is still to be substantiated [29–31].

7.8   Failure/Problems with the Spinal Component

Failure of the spinal component of CSE is more common with the needle-through-needle technique than with the separate needle technique. In the case of the needle-through-needle technique, failure of the spinal component can occur for a number of reasons (Fig. 7.6). A short spinal needle may not protrude far enough beyond the tip of the Tuohy needle to puncture the dura. On the other hand, a long needle may be more

Fig. 7.6 A short spinal needle may not protrude far enough beyond the tip of the Tuohy needle to puncture the dura. Deviation from the midline will also increase the epidural-dural distance and may result in the spinal needle missing the subarachnoid space laterally (adapted from Fig. 3.5 with permission)

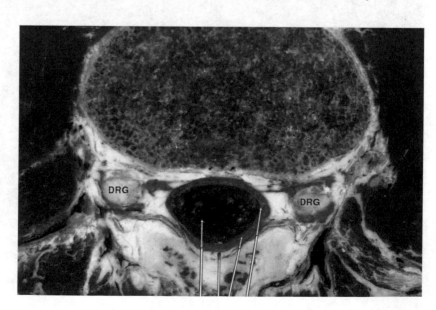

difficult to handle. Deviation from the midline will also increase the epidural-dural distance and may result in the spinal needle missing the subarachnoid space laterally. If "loss of resistance to saline" has been used to identify the epidural space, backflow of saline through the spinal needle may be mistaken for cerebrospinal fluid, which may contribute to the failure of the spinal component.

If problems are encountered with inserting an epidural catheter when the spinal dose has already been given, this may favor an uncontrolled sensory block spread before the anesthetist has had a chance to position the patient. For example, if the CSE is performed in the sitting position and the epidural catheter placement is delayed, there may be the risk of producing a saddle block. Furthermore, significant side effects of the subarachnoid block, such as hypotension, may occur at a time when the anesthetist's attention is centered on attempting to insert the epidural catheter.

To overcome these failure problems and to make more accurate identification of the epidural space, real-time ultrasonic scanning of the lumbar spine has been reported [32]. It provides an accurate reading of the location of the needle tip and facilitates the performance of combined spinal-epidural anesthesia (Fig. 7.7). Limitations of this technique have been discussed in Chap. 6.

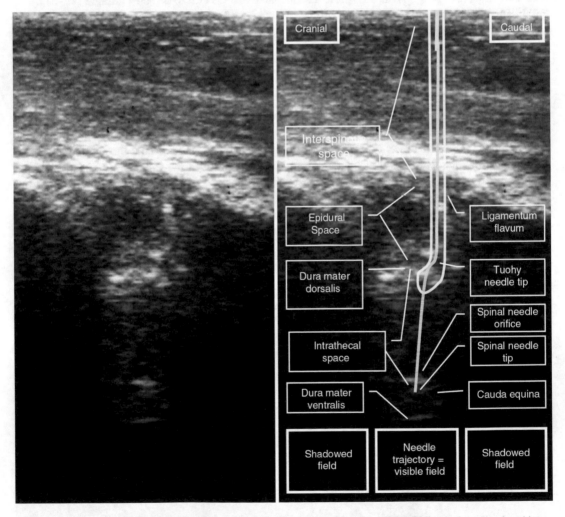

Fig. 7.7 Real-time ultrasound image with the Tuohy needle placed epidurally and the CSE spinal needle placed intrathecally. Localization of the needles and structures (from [32] with permission)

7.9 Epidural Volume Extension Technique

A low subarachnoid block can be extended significantly in a cephalad direction by an epidural "top-up" of 10 mL of normal saline given within 5 min of the subarachnoid block. This effect is known as epidural volume extension (EVE). The mechanism of this effect is probably related to compression of the subarachnoid space by the saline in the epidural space, which compresses the theca "squeezing" the cerebrospinal fluid, and resulting in more cephalad extensive spread of the subarachnoid block [33].

EVE allows CSE to be performed with small initial intrathecal doses of local anesthetic and, as saline is used for the epidural "top-ups," the total dose of local anesthetic used is reduced. EVE has been successfully used to provide anesthesia for elective cesarean section and may be associated with faster recovery of motor function in the postoperative period compared to single-shot spinal anesthesia [34]. EVE-induced sensory block augmentation has adequate documentation [35]; however, since EVE uses reduced intrathecal doses, it may be associated with a higher risk of inadequate anesthesia and an increased use of intraoperative analgesic supplementation [36].

Indeed it should be remembered that increasing the cephalad level of a sensory block does not necessarily mean providing an adequate, dense surgical block.

In addition one may speculate that a procedure such as EVE, which causes dural compression, may increase the pregnancy-induced dural compression. Active labor, by causing uterine contractions, may further increase epidural space pressure and enhance the effect of EVE.

7.10 Test Dose After CSE

When subarachnoid block is established before placing an epidural catheter, a conventional epidural "test dose" cannot be correctly interpreted and may be potentially dangerous by extending subarachnoid block [37].

In theory, the test dose could be delayed until subarachnoid block is regressing, but this interrupts analgesia and correct interpretation remains difficult if residual block persists. In alternative, the problem could be solved if separate-needle CSE is used and the epidural catheter is placed and tested before subarachnoid block, but this may be impractical.

For labor analgesia a test dose is deemed to be unnecessary if dilute solutions are used [6] and since 30 years ago there has been a general consensus that each labor analgesia bolus should be regarded as a test dose [38]. It is also important to consider that when therapeutic analgesic doses are used as a test dose, the total dose may be equivalent to the one used for subarachnoid anesthesia. Therefore, if the catheter is accidentally placed intrathecally, the mother will present sensory motor block and hemodynamic compromise similar to what may be observed after spinal anesthesia for cesarean section.

However, using an untested epidural catheter to extend an epidural block for an unplanned cesarean section, in a preexisting CSE labor analgesia, is a major issue in obstetric anesthesia. Problems with the test dose may lead to a greater reliance on negative aspiration tests to confirm epidural catheter placement.

However, when performing needle-through-needle CSE, fluid has been noted at the hub of the epidural needle or, very often, even within the correctly positioned epidural catheter [39]; therefore, all boluses injected into an epidural catheter after CSE should be of such a nature that unintentional subarachnoid administration will not be dangerous and neural block must be monitored rigorously after boluses.

References

1. Soresi AL. Episubdural anesthesia. Anesth Analg. 1937;16:306–10.
2. Curelaru I. Long duration subarachnoid anesthesia with continuous epidural blocks. Praktische Anaesthesie Wiederbelebung und Intensivtherapie. 1979;14:71–8.
3. Brownridge P. Epidural and subarachnoid analgesia for elective caesarean section. Anaesthesia. 1981;36:70.

4. Coates MB. Combined subarachnoid and epidural techniques [letter]. Anaesthesia. 1982;37:89–90.
5. Rawal N. Single segment combined subarachnoid and epidural block for cesarean section. Can Anaesth Soc J. 1986;33:254–5.
6. Collis RE, Baxandall ML, Srikantharajah ID, et al. Combined spinal epidural (CSE) analgesia: technique, management and outcome of 300 mothers. IJOA. 1994;3:75–81.
7. Tanaka N, Ohkubo S, Takasaki M. Evaluation of a lockable combined spinal-epidural device for use with needle-through-needle technique. Masui. 2004;53:173–7.
8. Eldor J, Brodsky V. Danger of metallic particles in the spinal-epidural spaces using the needle-through-needle approach(letter). Acta Anaesthesiol Scand. 1991;35:461.
9. Herman N, Molin J, Knape KG. No additional metal particle formation using the needle-through-needle combined spinal/epidural technique. Acta Anaesthesiol Scand. 1996;40:227–31.
10. Eldor J, Gozal Y, Guedj E, et al. Combined spinal-epidural anesthesia with a specialized needle. Reg Anesth. 1991;16:348–9.
11. Coombs DW. Multi-lumen epidural-spinal needle. U.S. Patent No. 4,808,157; 1989.
12. Stamenkovic D, Geric V, Djordjevic M, et al. Subarachnoid morphine, bupivacaine and fentanyl as part of combined spinal-epidural analgesia for low anterior resection. A prospective, randomized, double-blind clinical trial. Anaesth Intensive Care. 2009;37:552–60.
13. Cook TM. Combined spinal epidural techniques. Anaesthesia. 2000;55:42–64.
14. Dahl JB, Rosenberg J, Dirkes WE, et al. Prevention of postoperative pain by balanced analgesia. Br J Anaesth. 1990,64:518–20.
15. Vercauteren MP, Geernaert K, Vandeput DM, et al. Combined continuous spinal-epidural anaesthesia with a single interspace, double-catheter technique. Anaesthesia. 1993;48:1002–4.
16. Nikalls RWD, Dennison B. A modification of the combined spinal and epidural technique. Anaesthesia. 1984;39:935–6.
17. Katz J. Spinal and epidural anatomy. In: Katz J, editor. Atlas of regional anaesthesia. Norwalk: Appleton-Century-Crofts; 1985. p. 168–9.
18. Slattery PJ, Rosen M, Rees GAD. An aid to identification of the subarachnoid space with a 25-gauge needle. Anaesthesia. 1980;35:391.
19. Joshi GP, McCaroll MC. Evaluation of combined spinal-epidural anesthesia using two different techniques. Reg Anesth. 1994;19:169–74.
20. Casati A, D'Ambrosio A, De Negri P, et al. A clinical comparison between needle-through-needle and double-segment techniques for combined spinal and epidural anesthesia. RAPM. 1998;23:390–4.
21. Urmey WF, Stanton J, Sharrock NE. Combined spinal/epidural anesthesia for outpatient surgery-in reply. Anesthesiology. 1996;84:481–2.
22. Carter LC, Popat MT, Wallace DH. Epidural needle rotation and inadvertent dural puncture with the catheter. Anaesthesia. 1992;47:447–8.

23. Holstrom B, Rawal N, Axelson K, et al. Risk of catheter migration during combined spinal epidural block: percutaneous epiduroscopy study. Reg Anesth. 1995;80:747–53.
24. Angle PJ, Kronberg JE, Thompson DE, et al. Epidural catheter penetration of human dural tissue: in vitro investigation. Anesthesiology. 2004;100:1491–6.
25. Leach A, Smith GB. Subarachnoid spread of epidural local anesthetic following dural puncture. Anaesthesia. 1988;43:671–4.
26. Vartis A, Collier CB, Gatt SP. Potential intrathecal leakage of solutions injection into the epidural space following combined spinal epidural anaesthesia. Anaesth Intensive Care. 1998;26:256–61.
27. Beaubien G, Drolet P, Girard M, et al. Patient-controlled epidural analgesia with fentanyl-bupivacaine: influence of prior dural puncture. Reg Anesth Pain Med. 2000;25:254–8.
28. Bernards CM, Kopacz DJ, Michel MZ. Effect of needle puncture on morphine and lidocaine flux through the spinal meninges of the monkey in vitro: implications for combined spinal–epidural anesthesia. Anesthesiology. 1994;80:853–8.
29. Thomas JA, Pan PH, Harris LC, et al. Dural puncture with a 27-gauge Whitacre needle. Anesthesiology. 2005;103:1046–51.
30. Cappiello E, O'Rourke N, Segal S, et al. A randomized trial of dural puncture epidural technique. Anesth Analg. 2008;107:1646–51.
31. Chau A, Bibbo C, Huang CC, et al. Dural puncture epidural technique improves labor analgesia quality. Anesth Analg. 2017;124:560–9.
32. Grau T, Leipold W, Fatehi S, et al. Real-time ultrasonic observation of combined spina-epidural anaesthesia. EJA. 2004;21:25–31.
33. Takiguchi T, Okano T, Egawa H, et al. The effect of epidural saline injection on analgesic level during combined spinal and epidural anesthesia assessed clinically and myelographically. Anesth Analg. 1997;85:1097–100.
34. Lew E, Yeo SW, Thomas E. Combined spinal-epidural anesthesia using epidural volume extension leads to faster motor recovery after elective cesarean delivery: a prospective, randomized, double-blind study. Anesth Analg. 2004;983:810–4.
35. Tyagi A, Sharma CS, Kumari S, et al. Epidural volume extension: a review. Anaesth Intensive Care. 2012;40:604–13.
36. Loubert C, O'Brien PJ, Fernando R, et al. Epidural volume extension in combined spinal epidural anaesthesia for elective caesarean section: a randomized controlled trial. Anaesthesia. 2011;66:341–7.
37. Bickford Smith PJ. Cardiorespiratory arrest and combined spinal/epidural anaesthesia for caesarean section. Anaesthesia. 1994;49:83–4.
38. Van Zundert A, Vaes L, Soetens M, et al. Every dose in epidural analgesia for vaginal delivery can be a test dose. Anesthesiology. 1987;67:436–40.
39. Haridas RP. Cerebrospinal fluid leak with combined spinal epidural analgesia. Anesthesiology. 1997;87:A785.

The traditional contraindications to epidural block are skin infections at the site of puncture, coagulopathy, and sepsis, although these are not the only risk factors for spinal hematoma and abscess, and uncorrected maternal hypovolemia (hemorrhage). Particular precautions should be taken with patients with intracranial lesions and spinal malformations. Inadequate training and experience and patient refusal or inability to cooperate may be added to the list, but such a constraint applies to *any* treatment that is offered.

8.1 Skin and Soft-Tissue Alterations at the Site of the Puncture

8.1.1 Bacterial Infection

Localized skin infection at lumbar level, at the site of the puncture, is commonly included in the risk factors for epidural abscess and, therefore, it is usually considered to be an absolute contraindication to neuraxial anesthesia. However, there are no recommendations regarding the minimum distance between the puncture site and the site of infection.

8.1.2 Fungal Infection

8.1.2.1 Tinea (Pityriasis) Versicolor

Tinea (pityriasis) versicolor is a fungal infection caused by the dimorphic yeast Malassezia furfur and *Malassezia globosa*. This yeast is part of the normal skin flora and is largely considered to be of low pathogenicity. The organism resides in the stratum corneum and hair follicles. Incidence is greatest during adolescence and young adulthood. Manifestation of the rash only occurs when the yeast converts from the budding to the hyphal form. Heat and humidity play a significant role in this conversion. Other risk factors for conversion to the hyphal form include pregnancy, oral contraceptive usage, immunosuppression, malnutrition, burns, corticosteroid therapy, depressed cellular immunity, and genetic predisposition.

The typical presentation of tinea versicolor is that of multiple hypo- and hyperpigmented maculopapular lesions most commonly found over the chest, abdomen, and back. The rash is usually asymptomatic although it may be associated with pruritus.

In all cases it should be taken into account that (1) the absence of rash over a particular location in the affected patient does not ensure the organism's absence at the needle insertion site, (2) all patients have commensal organisms normally found on the skin, and (3) the presence of microorganisms is necessary, but not sufficient, to cause neuraxial infections.

Skin antisepsis is important: 2% chlorhexidine gluconate in 70% isopropyl alcohol penetrates five layers of dermis and has antifungal properties. Local anesthetics have antimicrobial activity against both bacteria and fungi as well. The anti-

© Springer Nature Switzerland AG 2020
G. Capogna, *Epidural Technique In Obstetric Anesthesia*,
https://doi.org/10.1007/978-3-030-45332-9_8

fungal properties of both the skin preparation and local anesthetic solution as well as the patient's intrinsic immunologic defenses likely contribute to a very low risk of neuraxial infections in parturients with tinea versicolor.

Keeping in mind that fungal infections affect only the superficial layers of the epidermis, after appropriate aseptic treatment, a skin incision at the puncture site may be used to advance the needle directly through the dermis, avoiding contamination of the deeper layers by the epidermis-infected cells.

8.1.3 Viral Infections

8.1.3.1 Pityriasis Rosea (Beta-Herpesvirus Infection)

Pityriasis rosea is an acute, self-healing, disease of the skin that begins with the appearance of a singular oval-shaped pink lesion followed by the eruption of numerous thin papules that spread symmetrically over the trunk in a distribution often referred to as a "Christmas tree" pattern (Fig. 8.1). It is commonly associated to general malaise, fever, headache, nausea, pruritus, arthralgias, and loss of appetite. On average, it has a median duration of 45 days and has a predominancy for the feminine gender and it may be seen in the obstetric population. Pityriasis rosea is a beta-herpesvirus infection and therefore potential treatments include topical steroids, oral antihistamines, acyclovir, and, when the disease is severe, phototherapy. The skin lesions of pityriasis rosea are not due to direct infection of skin cells, but rather occur as a reactive response to systemic viral replication [1] and therefore the risk for seeding the central nervous system (CNS) with virions from the skin may be less than that of patients with the active alpha-herpesvirus infection (such as the rare form of disseminate herpes zoster infection, in which the cutaneous lesions may be extended also to the dorsum), which replicate in epithelial cells during active infection.

Pityriasis rosea should be, however, considered a contraindication to regional anesthesia since there is no sufficient evidence of the risk of meningitis or encephalitis from blood to CNS

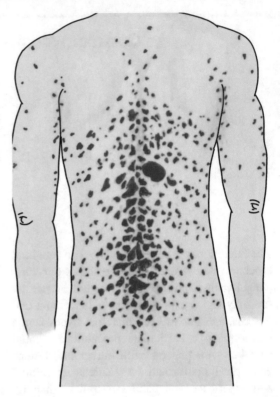

Fig. 8.1 The characteristic "Christmas tree" distribution of pityriasis rosea papules with herald patch

transmission when these patients are with active infection.

8.1.4 Tattoos

Increasingly women of child-bearing age have tattoos, frequently in the lumbar and sacral areas. Many pigments are not intended for use in humans and the tattoo artists are not regulated by national agencies. Some anesthesiologists avoid inserting an epidural needle through a tattoo on the lower back because of the fear of complications related to tattoo pigment debris introduced in the epidural space by the epidural needle.

Anonymous surveys of anesthesiologists reported no agreement about the provision of epidural analgesia for pregnant women with lower back tattoos; in one, 40% of respondents indicated that they would not perform the procedure, and 70% reported no agreed departmental policy for their management [2, 3].

Although the literature review reports no evidence of serious complications [4], a needle passed through a tattoo can entrap pigmented tissue fragments (cores) into the epidural or subarachnoid space. It is not clear if this may induce a risk of late neurological complications, related to an inflammatory or granulomatous response caused by metallic salts in tattoo pigment debris introduced in these spaces. The data regarding tissue coring and epidermoid tumor formation are reassuring, and it appears that the risk of their development after neuraxial procedures is likely to be extremely low, albeit currently unquantifiable.

To avoid this theoretical risk, the physician should try to avoid puncturing through the tattoo, either by selecting a different vertebral interspace or by using a paramedian approach or by finding a pigment-free skin spot within the area of the tattoo. When these options cannot be implemented, a superficial skin incision prior to needle insertion should prevent from coring tattoo pigment when entering the skin. Whatever the final choice, the technique to be implemented should be determined as early as the antenatal visit, after informed consent.

8.2   Systemic Infection: Febrile Patient

The risk of CNS infection may theoretically occur in any bacteremic patient. Metastatic infection from sources elsewhere may find a favorable growing place in an area predisposed to infection by mild trauma or irritation from an epidural needle or indwelling epidural catheter, and for this reason epidural analgesia or anesthesia is often considered contraindicated in the presence of systemic infection.

It is a common concern among anesthesiologists that administration of regional anesthesia to a febrile parturient may spread the infectious agent to the central nervous system and lead to neurological sequelae. However, to date no epidemiologic study has documented a causal relationship between dural puncture in the presence of bacteremia and the subsequent development

of complications such as meningitis and epidural abscess [5].

Provided that the infection is well under control with appropriate antibiotic therapy, the risk of an epidural nidus would seem to be remote and acceptable if epidural analgesia is indicated.

Administration of epidural anesthesia and short-term epidural catheterization is most likely safe in the parturient with chorioamnionitis without bacteremia or sepsis signs and treated with antibiotics [6, 7].

However, neuraxial blocks are generally contraindicated in obstetric sepsis, due to poor hemodynamic tolerance, probability of coagulopathy or thrombocytopenia, and risk of meningitis or epidural abscesses [8].

8.2.1   Systemic Viral Infections: HIV, Herpes Simplex, Herpes Zoster (Alpha Herpesvirus, HHV1, -2, and -3)

Concerns regarding the safety of epidural block in patients with HIV infection due to the fear of causing neurological sequelae through the needle trauma are balanced by the absence of a definite contraindication in a "relatively healthy" parturient [9]. Neuraxial anesthesia may be the anesthetic method of choice in pregnant women when compared with general anesthesia [10].

This is because it does not accelerate the neurological disease progression and because of the inherent risks of general anesthesia in these patients (esophageal and oropharyngeal disorders predisposing to regurgitation and aspiration, opportunistic lung infections, drug interactions, impact of general anesthesia on organs, liver or renal dysfunction, history of drug abuse). The indication of a blood patch with autologous blood after dural tap is considered to be safe, and it does not predispose the patient to neurological disease progression with a follow-up period of 2 years [11].

Viremia due to any virus from the herpesvirus family (herpes simplex virus 1 and 2, and herpes virus varicella-zoster) usually occurs during primary infection, followed by a neuronal persistence with ulterior virus reactivation. For this reason a safe distance between the puncture site and active lesions needs to be considered.

There are no maternal or neonatal infectious complications following neuraxial anesthetic techniques in pregnant women with active herpetic lesions, with the exception of an increased risk of herpes labialis (oral herpes) reactivation after the administration of epidural morphine [12].

8.3 Patients Receiving Anticoagulants

Guidelines for regional anesthesia management in the anticoagulated patient have been developed, well established, and regularly updated [13–17].

These guidelines are, however, based on case reports or cohort surveys and therefore the decision to perform spinal or epidural analgesia in an anticoagulated parturient is individually tailored according to the hematoma risk and the benefits of regional analgesia. Epidural block is usually contraindicated in the high-thrombotic-risk patients (mechanical heart valves, lupus, combined or antithrombin deficiency, arterial thrombosis, recent (<3 months) deep vein thrombosis, and a history of pregnancy or postpartum thrombosis). In these patients if antithrombotic drugs cannot be discontinued alternative analgesia should be chosen and explained to the parturient. In low-thrombotic-risk patients receiving anticoagulants to prevent placental vascular disease, anticoagulants should be stopped at the end of pregnancy and labor epidural analgesia can be performed after the anticoagulation period. For intermediate-risk patients, the coagulation status should be optimized and monitored to ensure normal hemostasis recovery at the time of epidural catheter placement and removal [15, 18].

Both the ASRA and the ESA [15, 16] recommend that with regard to UFH, if the dose is <5000 units twice a day no further testing is required before neuraxial anesthesia. Doses of >5000 units twice a day require documentation of a normal PTT before epidural placement. A

platelet count should also be checked to rule out heparin-induced thrombocytopenia if the patient has been receiving heparin for >4 days.

With LMWH no testing is required, but neuraxial anesthesia should be delayed by either 12 h or 24 h from the last injection of LMWH depending on whether the patient is receiving prophylactic or therapeutic doses of LMWH, respectively. If the patient has an epidural catheter placed, LMWH administration should be delayed for 4 h after catheter removal.

At the end of pregnancy, the cervical maturation and obstetrical conditions for inducing labor are the most important parameters guiding LMWH discontinuation and allowing labor analgesia. These obstetrical conditions must be strictly and frequently monitored to optimize the therapeutic strategy.

Although it is rare for a pregnant woman to be taking the newer oral anticoagulants, such as dabigatran or rivaroxaban, if a patient taking these medications is encountered, neuraxial block should be delayed by 5 and 3 days, respectively.

8.4 Disorders of Coagulation

8.4.1 Inherited Coagulation Disorders

Due to the low prevalence of inherited coagulation disorders, routine screening for inherited coagulation disorders is not recommended except in the case of a personal or immediate family history of bleeding. However, parturients who present with known disorders or bleeding history (mucocutaneous bleeding or menorrhagia) are at an increased risk of bleeding complications during pregnancy and childbirth [19].

There are no current recommendations on the mode of delivery for these patients and the presence of a bleeding disorder does not necessarily preclude normal spontaneous vaginal delivery with neuraxial analgesia.

Von Willebrand disease (VWD) is the most common inherited bleeding disorder in the general population. Spinal, epidural, and combined spinal-epidural anesthesia may be safely used in the type 1 disease [20–22]; however there is a general consensus that patients with normalized VWF:RCo, factor VIII, and VWF antigen concentrations are the best candidates for neuraxial anesthesia. The epidural catheter should be removed as soon after delivery as possible because factor concentrations decrease rapidly after delivery. If the catheter is maintained in situ after delivery, documentation of normal factor concentrations should be obtained before its removal.

Although hemophilia A and B (severe factor VIII and IX deficiency, respectively) are extremely rare in females, carrier status is much more common. The safe placement of neuraxial anesthesia in hemophilia carriers is well documented, both in pregnant and in nonpregnant patients [20], but where the patient is a known carrier, the factor concentrations of VIII/IX should be normalized before epidural placement.

8.4.2   Platelet Disorders

Among acquired disorders, platelet disorders are the most common hematological disorders during pregnancy. Almost all thrombocytopenia during pregnancy are related to one of the three causes: gestational thrombocytopenia, hypertensive disorders such as preeclampsia, or idiopathic thrombocytopenic purpura (ITP).

During gestational thrombocytopenia or ITP, the platelet count is usually stable while during preeclampsia the platelet count can rapidly change and therefore it is important to obtain serial platelet counts. In addition, the platelet function is typically normal in gestational thrombocytopenia and ITP, whereas it may be abnormal in severe preeclampsia and in this latter case it may be further complicated by hemolysis, elevated liver enzymes, and low platelet syndrome with coagulopathy. To my knowledge, there is only one case report in the literature of a parturient with preeclampsia with thrombocytopenia who developed an epidural hematoma, and in this case, she underwent a laminectomy and fully recovered [23].

At the present time there is no definition of the minimal platelet count below which it is unsafe to perform epidural anesthesia. Indeed, each patient must be individualized, and the physician must weigh the risks and benefits. A routine platelet count is not necessary in the otherwise-healthy parturient and should be done based on patient history, physical examination, and clinical signs. If the platelet count is found to be low it is important to confirm this finding because automated counters can be unreliable, especially at lower platelet counts. A manual count should be undertaken, because it is not uncommon to find that the platelets are clumping, and the count is really greater than calculated. Patient history and physical examination are key components when deciding whether to proceed with an epidural block in the parturient with thrombocytopenia. I will place an epidural catheter in a woman with a stable platelet count of 70,000–75,000 mm^{-3}. Generally speaking if there is any history of easy bruising or if the patient has evidence of petechiae or ecchymosis, epidural block should not be offered. If the patient has no bleeding history, then my general practice is to obtain at least one additional platelet count as close in time to epidural catheter placement as possible to ensure that it is not decreasing. This is especially important for disease processes that are dynamic, such as preeclampsia.

The etiology of thrombocytopenia and determining whether platelets are functioning adequately are the most important factors and a consultation with a hematologist may sometimes be needed. The risks of epidural placement vs. general anesthesia have to be individualized, and informed consent must be obtained.

If the decision is made to place an epidural catheter with a platelet count lower than 70,000^{-3}, soft-tipped catheters should be used to minimize trauma to epidural vessels, and the lowest concentration of local anesthetics should be used, in order to preserve motor function. The patient should be frequently examined (every 1–2 h) to assess the extent of the motor block, and these examinations should continue until after the anesthesia or analgesia has worn off and the catheter has been removed. In this way, if the patient develops a motor block out of proportion to what one would expect, the development of an epidural hematoma may be suspected and the patient must be assessed immediately with magnetic resonance imaging.

8.5   Intracranial Lesions

Parturients with intracranial lesions are often assumed to have increased intracranial pressure (ICP) and for this reason this condition is usually considered as a contraindication to neuraxial anesthesia due to the risk of herniation after an inadvertent dural puncture.

In order to understand the association between ICP and brain herniation, it is important to define intracranial compliance which is the relationship between the ICP and the volume of brain, cerebrospinal fluid (CSF), and blood within the cranium.

8.5.1   Fundamental Considerations

The brain (approximately 1400 mL of volume) is a relatively non-compressible structure.

The intracranial volume of CSF is approximately 150 mL and is contained in the cerebral ventricles and freely communicates back and forth within the extracranial subarachnoid space. CSF is reabsorbed in the arachnoid granulations, which then empty into the intracranial venous sinuses (which are non-compressible since they are located in the skull). The CSF system acts like a compressible cushion within and around the brain. Approximately 400–500 mL of new CSF is produced daily. Each of the intracranial and spinal compartments of the CSF system typically contains 150 mL of CSF, and the remainder is continuously reabsorbed. Normal CSF pressure ranges from 13 to 20 cm H_2O.

If the flow of CSF is impeded within or between the ventricles, "non-communicating" or "obstructive" hydrocephalus occurs. However an increased ventricular volume is not always associated with increased ICP (such as in the case of cerebral atrophy which causes dilation of the ventricles without an increase in ICP).

Hydrocephalus associated with increased ICP may be due to the impaired absorption of CSF (communicating hydrocephalus) or obstruction of the CSF flow (obstructive hydrocephalus). Parturients with non-communicating hydrocephalus are typically at greater relative risk of acute neurological deterioration after intentional or inadvertent dural puncture, than those with communicating hydrocephalus.

The normal cerebral blood volume is approximately 150 mL and is influenced by a variety of factors, including the degree of vasoconstriction.

Within the noncompliant bony skull, the total intracranial volume remains a constant, such that an increase in the volume of any one component causes a compensatory decrease in the volume of another (Monro–Kellie doctrine).

In normal subjects, magnetic resonance imaging of the brain shows that CSF shifts from the intracranial to the spinal subarachnoid space during cardiac systole. This phenomenon is a physiologic response to the corresponding increased brain-blood volume that occurs with each systolic contraction (homeostasis based on the Monro–Kellie doctrine). During diastole, CSF returns to the intracranial compartment. Therefore, physiologic alterations in cerebral blood volume result in a transient, well-tolerated increase in ICP followed by rapid re-equilibration, which does not compromise neurologic function [24–26].

The respiratory cycle also produces small, well-tolerated, oscillations of CSF pressure [27, 28].

Obesity and external abdominal compression result in decreased lumbar CSF volume [29], most likely due to the compression of the dural sac at the sites of intervertebral foramen in the abdomen.

During labor CSF pressure increases with contractions (mean rise 2.5 mmHg) [28] and this rise corresponds to an increase in central venous pressure, which persists even during sleep or total sensory block.

Injection of solutions into the lumbar epidural space compresses the dural sac, alters the compliance of the spinal subarachnoid space, and displaces CSF upward towards the cranium [30, 31].

Pregnancy and labor gradually increase baseline lumbar epidural pressure due to the space-occupying effect of the increased blood volume in distended epidural veins [32, 33].

Subjects with baseline-elevated ICP have more pronounced transient increases in ICP after epidural injection, than subjects with normal ICP. Significant (90%) but transient reduction in cerebral blood flow has been observed in an animal model with elevated ICP [30, 31].

Under normal conditions, the total intracranial volume is low enough so that, despite the routine physiologic perturbations associated with the cardiac and respiratory cycles, as well as those in pregnancy and vaginal delivery, the ICP fluctuates within the normal range and no neurologic consequences occur.

In the case of malignant tumors or conditions such as eclampsia, disruption of the blood-brain barrier frequently leads to vasogenic edema, which increases the extracellular water content, and subsequently the tissue volume, within the skull [34–37].

Abnormalities in intracranial blood vessels can also impact intracranial volume in a variety of ways. When vessel rupture occurs, it produces intracranial hemorrhage (subdural, intracerebral, or subarachnoid hemorrhage). Venous occlusion can also lead to secondary intracerebral hemorrhage. Any intracranial hemorrhage or other sudden increase in intracerebral blood volume has the potential to increase ICP by impeding the free flow of CSF either by exerting mass effect on the ventricular system or by causing thrombosis within the ventricles. Any of these circumstances can increase the risk of neurologic deterioration after neuraxial anesthesia.

8.5.2   The Impact of a Space-Occupying Lesion with or Without ICP

Of the intracranial tumors discovered during pregnancy due to detection of neurologic symptoms, gliomas represent the majority, followed by meningioma, and acoustic neuroma. Tumors such as meningiomas and pituitary adenomas can be hormone responsive and therefore may enlarge during pregnancy.

The effect of any space-occupying lesion on intracranial compliance is the most important factor to be evaluated in predicting the potential for neurologic deterioration from neuraxial anesthesia. The most relevant lesion characteristics are its location and size, the rapidity with which the overall brain tissue and volume have increased, and the presence of imaging evidence of preexisting fluid or tissue shifts or obstruction to CSF pathways.

To safely perform any dural puncture, there should be preservation of continuous flow of CSF and absence of a significant differential pressure between the intracranial and the intraspinal compartments. If a pressure differential exists, then loss of sufficient CSF volume throughout the dural puncture could force brain tissue to shift from one compartment to another. In addition, because there will most likely be some loss of lumbar CSF after a lumbar dural puncture, there should be sufficient remaining intracranial CSF so that CSF will shift to equalize the pressure rather than brain tissue.

However, a space-occupying lesion is not always associated with an increased ICP.

For example, if a primary brain tumor is located in a region which is remote from CSF pathways, and is of small-to-moderate size or grows slowly over time, it may cause little or no ventricular compression, and, therefore, have no impact on CSF flow. A sudden loss of lumbar CSF volume at the time of dural puncture will cause a transient pressure gradient across the foramen magnum. In this case, CSF rather than brain tissue will be displaced from the intracranial to the lumbar CSF compartment and there should be no herniation of brain tissue. Similarly, one would expect that in this patient with normal pre-procedure ICP, the transient increase in ICP associated with epidural injection would also be well tolerated [38–41].

Typically, these patients lack signs of increased ICP such as headache, nausea, vomiting, decreased alertness, recent seizure, hemiparesis, or pupillary abnormalities, or imaging evidence suggestive of increased ICP.

In contrast, if the intracranial lesion partially or completely obstructs the free flow of CSF, then the risk of brain herniation after intentional or accidental dural puncture is increased [42].

Lesions located at an anatomically narrowed segment of the ventricular system (near the third ventricle or cerebral aqueduct) or at the foramen magnum can place the parturient at significant risk of herniation. As the lesion grows, it displaces intracranial CSF caudally, or in the case of an obstruction to CSF outflow, it causes increased ventricular volume and hydrocephalus.

If the intracranial CSF has been exhausted and the lumbar CSF pressure suddenly drops from a dural puncture, then brain tissue itself will be displaced into the neighboring intracranial compartment or into the spinal canal (tonsillar herniation) and significant neurological deterioration typically ensues [43–46].

8.5.3   Arnold-Chiari Malformation

By definition, Arnold-Chiari malformations are structural defects in the cerebellum characterized by the downward displacement of the cerebellar tonsils at least 5 mm through the foramen magnum, sometimes leading to non-communicating hydrocephalus as a result of obstruction of CSF flow.

The most common form of this congenital disease is the type I, which is characterized by the above-described downward displacement of the cerebellar tonsils and which may be associated with cervical syringomyelia. Parturients with the most common form, type I, may be asymptomatic or may display symptoms, including headache, ataxia, and/ or sensorimotor impairments of the extremities.

Type II is associated with myelomeningoceles and both the cerebellar and brain stem tissue extend into the foramen magnum, resulting in episodic apnea, cranial nerve dysfunction, and upper extremity weakness. Type II is associated with hydrocephalus, syringomyelia, and spinal lumbar myelomeningocele. In type III there is further protrusion of the cerebellum and the brain stem into the foramen magnum and the spinal cord, resulting in severe neurologic dysfunction. Type III is associated with syringomyelia, tethered cord, and hydrocephalus. Type IV disease involves cerebellar hypoplasia. Successful surgical correction removes the obstruction but some of the associated anomalies, such as a tethered spinal cord, may persist and may represent important contraindications to neuraxial anesthesia. It may be possible to carefully proceed with a spinal or epidural analgesia or anesthesia in a parturient with an asymptomatic type I Chiari malformation since there are many reports documenting successful and uneventful spinal and epidural analgesia and anesthesia in these patients [47–49].

However, if the patient has an inadvertent large-gauge needle dural puncture and/or develops a persistent headache or other neurologic symptoms, an early epidural blood patch is recommended because a decrease in CSF pressure can cause further herniation of the cerebellar tonsils [50].

8.5.4   Pseudotumor Cerebri

Idiopathic or benign intracranial hypertension, also known as pseudotumor cerebri, is a common condition, in which increased ICP does not imply herniation risk after dural puncture. This disorder, usually occurring in obese women of childbearing age, is defined by increased ICP (>20 cm H_2O) with normal CSF composition and absence of a known underlying cause.

In these women there is no obstruction to CSF flow and no baseline differential pressure between the intracranial and spinal CSF compartments. Therefore, a sudden drop in CSF volume during lumbar dural puncture will be rapidly accommodated by caudal flow of CSF and should not result in brain shift or herniation.

Indeed the therapy for this disease includes serial lumbar punctures for deliberate removal of large volumes of CSF, coupled with weight control, diuretics, and steroids. Neuraxial anesthesia may be used effectively for parturients with benign intracranial hypertension with or without shunts. However the use of 5 mL incremental, slow, boluses of epidural solution is suggested which may be better tolerated in symptomatic patients who might otherwise experience exacerbation of their symptoms due to the predelivery increase in ICP [51–57].

8.5.5 Individual Patient Assessment

As with all high-risk parturients, ensuring antepartum anesthesia consultation and multidisciplinary planning is extremely important in pregnant patients with intracranial pathology. The decisional algorithm to assess the risks of neuraxial anesthesia in parturients with space-occupying lesions is reported in Fig. 8.2, and helps to provide the framework for informed consultative questions [58].

There is no evidence of danger to fetal safety owing to the performance of maternal brain magnetic resonance imaging and therefore this exam should not be withheld during pregnancy if needed [59].

Parturients at high risk of herniation from a dural puncture are those with lesions that compress normal brain tissue and cause it to shift across the midline or downward, with or without obstruction to the flow of CSF. Parturients with space-occupying lesions that have no mass effect, hydrocephalus, or clinical or imaging findings suggestive of increased ICP are likely to have minimal to no increased risk of herniation from a dural puncture. A careful and multidisciplinary evaluation of this type of parturients not only permits appropriate low-risk candidates to benefit from the advantages of neuraxial anesthesia, but also allows proper preparation for general anesthesia for high-risk parturients when needed.

8.6 Spina Bifida

Spina bifida describes a variety of congenital abnormalities that arise as a result of failed closure of the neural tube. It is categorized as spina bifida cystica, which may include meningocele, myelomeningocele, rachischisis, and anencephaly and spina bifida occulta, which includes a wide range of minor defects. Although the spina bifida cystica is a very rare condition, the spina bifida occulta ranges from 10 to 50% of the adult population if its frequency is based on the presence of defects observed in the vertebral spinous processes and lamina [60, 61].

In addition, early repair of meningoceles and myelomeningoceles and advance in treatment of complications have resulted in an increasing number of patients with spina bifida cystica reaching childbearing age.

8.6.1 Spina Bifida Occulta

This is a relatively frequent condition, mostly at low lumbar and sacral level, which in most cases consists of isolated bony arch abnormalities often associated with posterior disc herniation. Epidural anesthesia is not contraindicated; the only recommendation is to perform the block at a site remote from the level of the anomaly. Supporting ligaments, specifically the interspi-

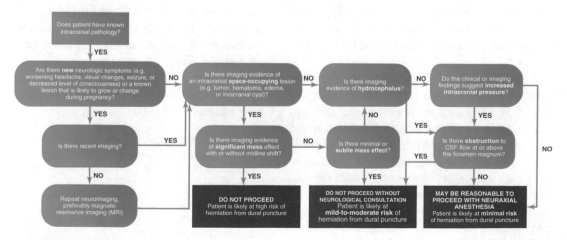

Fig. 8.2 The decisional algorithm to assess the risks of neuraxial anesthesia in parturients with space-occupying lesions (modified from [58])

nous ligament and the ligamentum flavum, may be abnormal at the level of the lesion, resulting in an increased potential for accidental dural puncture. The epidural space may also be discontinuous across the lesion, and inadequate or failed block may result.

Dimpling of the skin or a hairy patch at the base of the spine may be present in up to 70 % of the patients with cord abnormalities, of which only 30 % are symptomatic [38].

In these cases magnetic resonance imaging is recommended to exclude the presence of a tethered spinal cord or other possible cord abnormalities, after which it is acceptable to perform regional anesthesia at a level not affected by the abnormality.

8.6.2 Spina Bifida Cystica

The majority of spina bifida cystica patients are operated on in the first 24 h of life and improved surgical techniques allow the closure of large defects. Most patients develop hydrocephalus but not all require shunts to be placed. Associated abnormalities of the gastrointestinal, skeletal, cardiac, and renal systems may affect development. Progressive spinal deformities are observed in up to 90% of patients, with findings of scoliosis, kyphosis, and lordosis. Regional anesthesia is not contraindicated in patients with fixed neurologic deficits or previous spinal surgery, but it may be technically more difficult to perform. In these patients there is an increased risk of accidental dural puncture and incomplete blocks.

Spina bifida may be associated with another very rare condition, the tethered cord syndrome (Fig. 8.3). Clinically, the importance of this syndrome lies in the greater potential for direct spinal cord trauma while performing regional anesthesia, due to the low-lying conus medullaris. The syndrome may not be symptomatic until the precipitating event, such as childbirth, occurs and regional anesthesia may be implicated. Epidural may be safer than spinal anesthesia because of the low fixed cord, but the risk of epidural anesthesia in this group of patients is unknown.

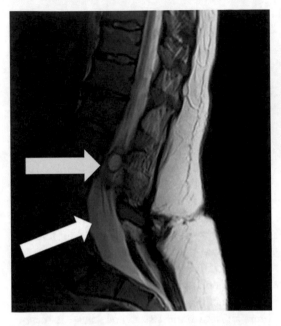

Fig. 8.3 T2-weighted sagittal image showing hydrosyringomyelia of the distal cord at the level of L1 (yellow arrow) and cord tethering at S1 (white arrow) (from [62] with permission)

There is still no consensus whether all patients with spina bifida should have an MRI scan when regional analgesia/anesthesia is planned. In theory any patient with spina bifida including spina bifida occulta may have a tethered cord even where no neurological symptoms are elicited [62, 63].

However, considering spina bifida as a relative or absolute contraindication to regional anesthesia and to use general anesthesia instead, it must be remembered that it is not without risk as several cases of difficult and failed intubations have been described [64].

References

1. Watanabe T, Kawamura T, Jacob SE, et al. Pityriasis rosea is associated with systemic active infection with both human herpesvirus-7 and human herpesvirus-6. J Invest Dermatol. 2002;119:793–7.
2. Sleth JC, Guillot B, Kluger N. Lumbar tattoos and neuraxial anesthesia in obstetrics: practice survey in Languedoc-Roussillon, France. Ann Fr Anesth Reanim. 2010;29:397–401.
3. Gaspar A, Serrano N. Neuraxial blocks and tattoos: a dilemma? Arch Gynecol Obstet. 2010;282:255–60.

4. Welliver D, Welliver M, Carroll T, et al. Lumbar epidural catheter placement in the presence of low back tattoos: a review of the safety concerns. ANA J. 2010;78:197–201.

5. Segal S, Carp H, Chestnut DH. Fever and infection. In: Chestnut DH, editor. Obstetric anesthesia: principles and practice. St. Louis: Mosby; 1999. p. 711–24.

6. Bader AM, Datta S, Gilbertson L, et al. Regional anesthesia in women with chorioamnionitis. Reg Anesth. 1992;17:84–6.

7. Goodman EJ, DeHorta E, Taguiam JM. Safety of spinal and epidural anesthesia in parturients with chorioamnionitis. Reg Anesth. 1996;21:436–41.

8. Elton RJ, Chaudari S. Sepsis in obstetrics. Br J Anaesth Educ. 2015;15:259–64.

9. Hughes SC, Dailey PA, Landers D, et al. Parturients infected with human immunodeficiency virus and regional anesthesia. Clinical and immunologic response. Anesthesiology. 1995;82:32–7.

10. Evron S, Glezerman M, Harow E, et al. Human immunodeficiency virus: anesthetic and obstetric considerations. Anesth Analg. 2004;98:503–11.

11. Tom DJ, Gurevich SJ, Shapiro HM, et al. Epidural blood patch in the HIV-positive patient: review of clinical experience. Anesthesiology. 1992;76:943–7.

12. Bauchat JR. Focused review: neuraxial morphine and oral herpes reactivation in the obstetric population. Anesth Analg. 2010;111:1238–41.

13. Bates SM, Greer IA, Middeldorp S, et al. VTE, thrombophilia, antithrombotic therapy, and pregnancy: antithrombotic therapy and prevention of thrombosis, 9th ed: American College of Chest Physicians evidence-based clinical practice guidelines. Chest. 2012;141(2 Suppl):e691S–736S.

14. Benhamou D, Mignon A, Aya G, et al. Prophylaxis of thromboembolic complications in obstetrics and gynaecology. Ann Fr Anesth Reanim. 2005;24:911–20.

15. Horlocker TT, Wedel DJ, Rowlingson JC, et al. Regional anesthesia in the patient receiving antithrombotic or thrombolytic therapy: American Society of Regional Anesthesia and Pain Medicine evidence-based guidelines (third edition). Reg Anesth Pain Med. 2010;35:64–101.

16. Gogarten W, Vandermeulen E, Van Aken H, et al. Regional anaesthesia and antithrombotic agents: recommendations of the European Society of Anaesthesiology. European Society of Anaesthesiology. Eur J Anaesthesiol. 2010;27:999–1015.

17. Butwick AJ, Carvalho B. Neuraxial anesthesia in obstetric patients receiving anticoagulant and antithrombotic drugs. Int J Obstet Anesth. 2010;19:193–201.

18. Hunt BJ, Gattens M, Khamashta M, et al. Thromboprophylaxis with unmonitored intermediate-dose low molecular weight heparin in pregnancies with a previous arterial or venous thrombotic event. Blood Coagul Fibrinolysis. 2003;14:735–9.

19. Dunkley SM, Russell SJ, Rowell JA, et al. A consensus statement on the management of pregnancy and delivery in women who are carriers of or have bleeding disorders. Med J Aust. 2009;191:460–3.

20. Choi S, Brull R. Neuraxial techniques in obstetric and non-obstetric patients with common bleeding diatheses. Anesth Analg. 2009;109:648–60.

21. Amorde R, Patel S, Pagel P. Management of labour and delivery of a patient with von Willebrand disease type 2 A. Int Anesthesiol Clin. 2011;49:74–80.

22. Kadir RA, Lee CA, Sabin CA, et al. Pregnancy in women with von Willebrand's disease or factor XI deficiency. Br J Obstet Gynaecol. 1998;105:314–21.

23. Lao TT, Halpern SH, MacDonald D, et al. Spinal subdural haematoma in a parturient after attempted epidural anaesthesia. Can J Anaesth. 1993;40:340–5.

24. Alperin NJ, Lee SH, Loth F, et al. MR-intracranial pressure (iCP): a method to measure intra-cranial elastance and pressure noninvasively by means of MR imaging: baboon and human study. Radiology. 2000;217:877–85.

25. Linninger AA, Xenos M, Zhu DC, et al. Cerebrospinal fluid flow in the normal and hydrocephalic human brain. IEEE Trans Biomed Eng. 2007;54:291–302.

26. Oldfield EH, Muraszko K, Shawker TH, et al. Pathophysiology of syringomyelia associated with Chiari I malformation of the cerebellar tonsils. Implications for diagnosis and treatment. J Neurosurg. 1994;80:3–15.

27. Friese S, Hamhaber U, Erb M, et al. B-waves in cerebral and spinal cerebrospinal fluid pulsation measurement by magnetic resonance imaging. J Comput Assist Tomogr. 2004;28:255–62.

28. Hopkins EL, Hendricks CH, Cibils LA. Cerebrospinal fluid pressure in labor. Am J Obstet Gynecol. 1965;93:907–16.

29. Hogan QH, Prost R, Kulier A, et al. Magnetic resonance imaging of cerebrospinal fluid volume and the influence of body habitus and abdominal pressure. Anesthesiology. 1996;84:1341–9.

30. Grocott HP, Mutch WA. Epidural anesthesia and acutely increased intracranial pressure. Lumbar epidural space hydrodynamics in a porcine model. Anesthesiology. 1996;85:1086–91.

31. Hilt H, Gramm HJ, Link J. Changes in intracranial pressure associated with extradural anaesthesia. Br J Anaesth. 1986;58:676–80.

32. Bromage PR. Continuous lumbar epidural analgesia for obstetrics. Can Med Assoc J. 1961;85:1136–40.

33. Galbert MW, Marx GF. Extradural pressures in the parturient patient. Anesthesiology. 1974;40:499–502.

34. Fox MW, Harms RW, Davis DH. Selected neurologic complications of pregnancy. Mayo Clin Proc. 1990;65:1595–618.

35. Crosby ET, Preston R. Obstetrical anaesthesia for a parturient with preeclampsia, HeLLP syndrome and acute cortical blindness. Can J Anaesth. 1998;45:452–9.

36. Schwartz RB, Feske SK, Polak JF, et al. Preeclampsia-eclampsia: clinical and neuroradiographic correlates and insights into the pathogenesis of hypertensive encephalopathy. Radiology. 2000;217:371–6.

37. Apollon KM, Robinson JN, Schwartz RB, et al. Cortical blindness in severe preeclampsia: computed

tomography, magnetic resonance imaging, and single-photon-emission computed tomography findings. Obstet Gynecol. 2000;95:1017–9.

38. May AE, Fombon FN, Francis S. UK registry of high-risk obstetric anaesthesia: report on neurological disease. Int J Obstet Anesth. 2008;17:31–6.

39. Finfer SR. Management of labour and delivery in patients with intracranial neoplasms. Br J Anaesth. 1991;67:784–7.

40. Terauchi M, Kubota T, Aso T, et al. Dysembryoplastic neuroepithelial tumor in pregnancy. Obstet Gynecol. 2006;108:730–2.

41. Chang LY, Carabuena JM, Camann W. Neurologic issues and obstetric anesthesia. Semin Neurol. 2011;31:374–84.

42. Gower DJ, Baker AL, Bell WO, et al. Contraindications to lumbar puncture as defined by computed cranial tomography. J Neurol Neurosurg Psychiatry. 1987;50:1071–4.

43. Beni-Adani L, Pomeranz S, Flores I, et al. Huge acoustic neurinomas presenting in the late stage of pregnancy. Treatment options and review of literature. Acta Obstet Gynecol Scand. 2001;80:179–84.

44. Boker A, Ong BY. Anesthesia for cesarean section and posterior fossa craniotomy in a patient with von Hippel-Lindau disease. Can J Anaesth. 2001;48:387–90.

45. Mamelak AN, Withers GJ, Wang X. Choriocarcinoma brain metastasis in a patient with viable intrauterine pregnancy. Case report. J Neurosurg. 2002;97:477–81.

46. Citerio G, Andrews PJ. Intracranial pressure. Part two: clinical applications and technology. Intensive Care Med. 2004;30:1882–5.

47. Landau R, Giraud R, Delrue V, et al. Spinal anesthesia for cesarean delivery in a woman with a surgically corrected type I Arnold-Chiari malformation. Anesth Analg. 2003;97:253–5.

48. Sicuranza GB, Steinberg P, Figueroa R. Arnold-Chiari malformation in a pregnant woman. Obstet Gynecol. 2003;102:1191–4.

49. Chantigian RC, Koehn MA, Ramin KD, et al. Chiari I malformation in parturients. J Clin Anesth. 2002;14:201–5.

50. Dewan DM. Chiari I malformation presenting as recurrent spinal headache. Anesth Analg. 1992;75:1025–6.

51. Alperin N, Ranganathan S, Bagci AM, et al. MRI evidence of impaired CSF homeostasis in obesity-associated idiopathic intracranial hypertension. Am J Neuroradiol. 2013;34:29–34.

52. Aly EE, Lawther BK. Anaesthetic management of uncontrolled idiopathic intracranial hypertension during labour and delivery using an intrathecal catheter. Anaesthesia. 2007;62:178–81.

53. Kaul B, Vallejo MC, Ramanathan S, et al. Accidental spinal analgesia in the presence of a lumboperitoneal shunt in an obese parturient receiving enoxaparin therapy. Anesth Analg. 2002;95:441–3.

54. Heckathorn J, Cata JP, Barsoum S. Intrathecal anesthesia for cesarean delivery *via* a subarachnoid drain in a woman with benign intracranial hypertension. Int J Obstet Anesth. 2010;19:109–11.

55. Bedson CR, Plaat F. Benign intracranial hypertension and anaesthesia for caesarean section. Int J Obstet Anesth. 1999;8:288–90.

56. Bédard JM, Richardson MG, Wissler RN. Epidural anesthesia in a parturient with a lumboperitoneal shunt. Anesthesiology. 1999;90:621–3.

57. Kim K, Orbegozo M. Epidural anesthesia for cesarean section in a parturient with pseudotumor cerebri and lumboperitoneal shunt. J Clin Anesth. 2000;12:213–5.

58. Leffert LR, Schwamm LH. Neuraxial anesthesia in parturients with intracranial pathology. Anesthesiology. 2013;119:703–18.

59. Klein JP, Hsu L. Neuroimaging during pregnancy. Semin Neurol. 2011;31:361–73.

60. Farine D, Jackson U, Portale A, et al. Pregnancy complicated by maternal spina bifida. J Reprod Med. 1988;33:323–6.

61. Avrahami E, Frishman E, Fridman Z, et al. Spina bifida occulta of S1 is not an innocent finding. Spine (Phila Pa 1976). 1994;19:12–5.

62. Murphy CJ, Stanley E, Kavanagh E, et al. Spinal dysraphisms in the parturient: implications for perioperative anaesthetic care and labour analgesia. Int J Obstet Anesth. 2015;24:252–63.

63. Roberts ND, May AE. Regional anaesthesia and spina bifida. Int J Obstet Anesth. 2002;11:12.

64. Anderson KJ, Quinlan MJ, Popat M, et al. Failed intubation in a parturient with spina bifida. Int J Obstet Anesth. 2000;9:64–8.

Complications

Only the complications due to the epidural technique will be described in this chapter.

Please refer to the standard textbooks for the complications due to the solutions injected, such as local anesthetic toxicity, total spinal anesthesia, etc.

9.1 Accidental Dural Puncture and Dural Puncture Headache

"I had a feeling of very strong pressure on my skull and became rather dizzy when I stood up rapidly from my chair. All these symptoms vanished at once when I lay down flat, but returned when I stood up. ... I was forced to take to bed and remained there for nine days, because all the manifestations recurred as soon as I got up. ... The symptoms finally resolved nine days after the lumbar puncture." This is the first description of consequences of dural puncture, made in 1898 by August Bier and his assistant, Dr. August Hildebrandt, who performed experiments with cocainization of the spinal cord on themselves.

Accidental dural puncture is of greatest concern in the obstetric anesthesia setting, since more than half of all parturients who experience an inadvertent dural puncture with an epidural needle will eventually develop headache symptoms, which may be associated with chronic headache and back pain [1, 2].

9.1.1 Pathophysiology

It is commonly agreed that PDPH is due to the loss of cerebrospinal fluid (CSF) through a persistent leak in the dura. However, the cellular arachnoid mater (containing frequent tight junctions and occluding junctions) is perhaps more important than the more permeable and acellular dura mater in the generation of symptoms.

The arachnoid membrane may exhibit tissue closure in relation to the dura because its main function is to act as a barrier; therefore, it may lack the elastic properties of the dural layer. The arachnoid layer limits the escape of fluid, so the amount of CSF lost through the punctured orifice is likely to be related to the speed of closure of the arachnoid lesion rather than to the dural one [3–7] (Fig. 9.1).

The term meningeal puncture headache (MPH) has therefore been proposed as an alternative to postdural puncture headache (PDPH), and this calls into question the interpretation of studies published in the past which examined isolated dura mater in vitro.

The actual mechanism by which CSF hypotension generates headache is currently attributed to a bimodal mechanism involving both loss of intracranial support and compensatory cerebral vasodilation. Reduced support due to CSF loss is thought to allow the brain to drop into the upright position, resulting in traction and pressure on pain-sensitive structures within the cranium (dura, cranial nerves, bridging veins, and venous sinuses). Adenosine-

© Springer Nature Switzerland AG 2020
G. Capogna, *Epidural Technique In Obstetric Anesthesia*,
https://doi.org/10.1007/978-3-030-45332-9_9

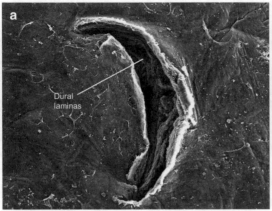 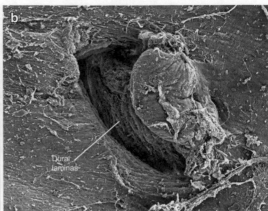

Fig. 9.1 (a) Dura-arachnoid lesion produced by 17G Tuohy needle. Internal surface of human dural sac (arachnoid layer). Scanning electron microscopy. Magnification: (a) ×50; (b) ×50 (from Reina M.A., López A., van Zundert A.A.J., De Andrés J.A. (2015) Ultrastructure of Dural Lesions Produced in Lumbar Punctures. In: Reina M., De Andrés J., Hadzic A., Prats-Galino A., Sala-Blanch X., van Zundert A. (eds) Atlas of Functional Anatomy for Regional Anesthesia and Pain Medicine. Springer, Cham with permission). (b) Dura-arachnoid lesion produced by 17G Tuohy needle. External surface of human dural sac (external dural laminas). Scanning electron microscopy. Magnification: (a) ×50; (b) ×400 (from Reina MA, Castedo J, López A. Cefalea pospunción dural. Ultraestructura de las lesiones durales y agujas espinales usadas en las punciones lumbares. Rev. Arg Anestesiol. 2008; 66:6–26 with permission by Elsevier)

mediated vasodilation may occur secondary to diminished intracranial CSF (in accordance with the Monro-Kellie hypothesis, which states that intracranial volume must remain constant) and reflexively secondary to traction on intracranial vessels. Multiple neural pathways are involved in generating the symptoms of PDPH. These include the ophthalmic branch of the trigeminal nerve in frontal head pain, cranial nerves IX and X in occipital pain, and cervical nerves in neck and shoulder pain. Nausea is attributed to vagal stimulation. Auditory and vestibular symptoms are secondary to the direct communication between the CSF and the perilymph via the cochlear aqueduct, which results in decreased perilymphatic pressures in the inner ear and an imbalance between the endolymph and perilymph. Significant visual disturbances are thought to represent a transient palsy of the nerves supplying the extraocular muscles of the eye.

9.1.2 Clinical Presentation and Characteristics

Onset of symptoms is generally delayed, with headache usually beginning 12–48 h and rarely more than 5 days following meningeal puncture [8].

The essential feature of PDPH is its postural nature, with headache symptoms worsening in the upright position and relieved, or at least improved, with recumbency. The International Headache Society (IHS) diagnostic criteria [9] further describe this positional quality as worsening within 15 min of sitting or standing and improving within 15 min after lying. Headache, whose severity varies considerably among patients, is always bilateral, with a distribution that is frontal (25%), occipital (27%), or both (45%). There is no standardized severity scale, but Lybecker proposed evaluating the headache intensity using a 10-point analog scale, with 1–3 classified as mild, 4–6 as moderate, and 7–10 as severe, also according to restriction in physical activity, degree of confinement to bed, and presence of associated symptoms [9].

The IHS criteria for PDPH require that headache be accompanied by at least one of the following symptoms [9]: neck stiffness, tinnitus, hypoacusia, photophobia, and nausea. However, these criteria cannot be considered as absolute, as many patients suffer from PDPH in the absence of any symptoms apart from the headache itself. Usually, the more severe the headache, the more likely it is to be accompanied by associated symptoms.

The most common associated symptoms are nausea, pain, and stiffness in the neck and shoulders. Uncommonly, patients may experience auditory or visual symptoms that can be unilateral, and the risk for either appears to be directly related to the needle size.

9.1.3   Risk Factors

The patient characteristic having the greatest impact on the risk of PDPH is age, the incidence declining over time. Gender is also a significant risk factor, females having approximately twice the risk when compared with males. Pregnancy has traditionally been regarded as a risk factor but this may be simply due to the fact that the pregnant population is a young female cohort with a relatively high incidence of inadvertent dural puncture with a large needle. Pushing during the second stage of labor may promote the loss of CSF through the hole in the meninges, and may increase the risk of PDPH following inadvertent dural puncture [10].

As described for spinal needles, meningeal puncture with larger epidural needles is associated with a higher incidence of PDPH, more severe headaches, more associated symptoms, a longer duration of symptoms, and a greater need for definitive treatment measures [11].

Very important factors in the development of PDPH are also the experience, the comfort, and the skill of the operator. Repeated number of punctures, inexperience, and fatigue play a major role in determining the incidence of accidental dural puncture during an epidural procedure [12].

9.1.4   Prevention and Prophylaxis

Unfortunately the overall quality of evidence for preventive measures is generally weak.

Ultrasound can decrease the number of needle passes required for epidural procedures but its potential to reduce the incidence of inadvertent dural puncture and therefore PDPH is still not defined. Bed rest and aggressive oral and intravenous hydration continue to be believed as one of the major prophylactic measures even if there is no evidence to support this common practice [13].

The risk of PDPH following ADP can be reduced by using the smallest feasible epidural needle [11].

Subarachnoid saline, intravenous cosyntropin, intrathecal epidural catheters, epidural saline, epidural opiates, and prophylactic epidural blood patch are sometimes used as prophylactic measures but none of these maneuvers are supported by strong scientific evidence [14, 15].

Among the most important preventive measures I should like to emphasize is a good knowledge of lumbar anatomy together with a carefully performed technique. It is well known that the inner surface of the ligamentum flavum is separated from the external surface of the dural sac by the epidural fat occupying the posterior epidural space. However, at the most lateral parts of the epidural space, where there is no epidural fat, the ligamentum flavum directly contacts the dural sac and this area is particularly at risk for inadvertent dural puncture [16]. If by chance the epidural needle is inserted in this area, the anesthesiologist should have the ability and the expertise to place the needle in the epidural space with a minimum extension without puncturing the dura (Fig. 9.2). Extension is defined as the distance the needle tip goes beyond the ligamentum flavum into the epidural space: the less the extension, the less likely the dural puncture will be, especially in that lateral area where the ligamentum flavum directly contacts the dural sac.

9.1.5   Diagnostic Evaluation

While numerous clinical variations have been reported, most cases of PDPH have a history of known or possible meningeal puncture, delayed onset of symptoms (but within 48 h), and bilateral postural headache (possibly accompanied by associated symptoms if moderate or severe). Fortunately, a careful history with a brief consideration of other possible diagnoses is usually all that is necessary to differentiate PDPH from other causes of headache. Although headache following dural puncture will naturally be sus-

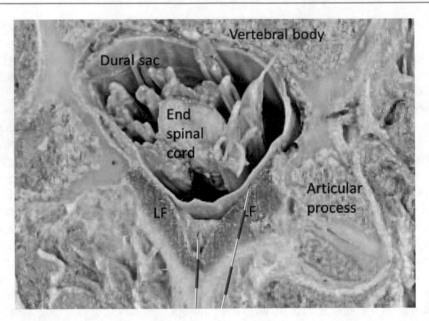

Fig. 9.2 Transverse section of human lumbar spine at L1 vertebral level (*LF* ligamentum flavum). At the most lateral parts of the epidural space, where there is no epidural fat, the ligamentum flavum directly contacts the dural sac and this area is particularly at risk for accidental dural puncture. Especially in this area, if the bevel of a Tuohy epidural needle is no longer than a few millimeters, the sooner the physician stops the advancement of the needle once it has entered the epidural space (and therefore less epidural needle coming out of the ligamentum flavum), the less likely an accidental dural puncture is to occur (modified from [16] with permission)

pected to be PDPH, it remains critical to rule out other causes.

A number of other benign etiologies are possible: nonspecific headache, tension-type headache, exacerbation of chronic headache, hypertensive headache, pneumoencephalus, sinusitis, drug-related side effects (such as caffeine withdrawal), and spontaneous intracranial hypotension. Serious causes of headache are rare but must be excluded: meningitis, subdural hematoma, subarachnoid hemorrhage, preeclampsia and eclampsia, and intracranial venous thrombosis.

A high index of suspicion should be maintained especially when typical PDPH progresses but loses its postural component.

9.1.6   Treatment

Once a diagnosis of PDPH has been made, patients should be provided with a straightforward explanation of the presumed etiology, told the anticipated natural course, and given a realistic assessment of treatment options.

Unfortunately there isn't any high-quality evidence supporting many commonly used forms of conservative and pharmacological methods of treatment of obstetric PDPH. As a possible example, this is the treatment suggested by the Obstetric Anaesthetists' Association (UK) who set up a working group to review the literature and produce evidence-based guidelines for management of obstetric postdural puncture headache [17]:

– Bed rest may reduce the intensity of symptoms, but prolonged bed rest is not recommended as it may increase the risk of thromboembolic complications.
– Thromboprophylaxis should be considered for women whose mobility is reduced due to PDPH.
– Encourage fluid intake to maintain adequate hydration.

- Offer simple oral analgesia such as paracetamol, weak opioids, and NSAIDs if not contraindicated.
- Stronger opioids such as morphine or oxycodone may be offered but treatment should usually be limited to <72-h duration.
- Caffeine may be offered but limited to 24-h duration, with a maximum dose of 900 mg (200 mg maximum in breastfeeding women).
- Offer an epidural blood patch (EBP) when symptoms affect daily living and care of the baby.

Although considered by many anesthesiologists as the gold standard for the treatment of obstetric PDPH, high-quality evidence on the management of an epidural blood patch (EBP) is limited [18].

The procedure itself has been well described and consists of the sterile injection of fresh autologous blood near the previous dural puncture.

The mechanism of action of the EBP, while not entirely elucidated, appears to be related to the ability to stop further CSF loss by the formation of a clot over the defect in the meninges as well as a tamponade effect with cephalad displacement of CSF (the "epidural pressure patch"). The appropriate role of the EBP in individual situations will depend on multiple factors, including the duration and severity of headache and associated symptoms, type and gauge of original needle used, and patient wishes.

Unfortunately, various aspects of the procedure, such as its efficacy, optimum timing, and duration of the supine position following the patch, are still not well defined. The balance of the risks of an EBP versus the potential consequences of non-interventional management is not fully understood [18].

Early reports of the EBP frequently cited high success rates but often did not include a strict definition of "success," had little or no follow-up, and failed to consider the influence of such confounding factors as needle size and tip design, severity of symptoms, or natural history of PDPH. The true efficacy of the EBP procedure is now known to be significantly lower than once thought [19].

Before hospital discharge, women who have experienced dural puncture with an epidural needle or PDPH should be given information on symptoms that require further medical assessment and information about who they should contact and what arrangements should be made for appropriate follow-up after discharge from hospital.

9.2 Accidental Subdural and Intradural Puncture

Significant uncertainty exists regarding the issue of an accidental injection of local anesthetic into the region commonly referred to as "subdural space" during attempted epidural block, particularly in obstetric patients. As most cases are suspected but not investigated, the real incidence is unknown since anatomical diagnosis is rarely made.

Most of the reported cases of accidental subdural block have been in obstetric patients receiving neuraxial analgesia for labor with a reported incidence varying from 0.8 to 0.02% depending on the criteria used to make the diagnosis due, in turn, to the large variability of presentation [20, 21].

9.2.1 Anatomical Basis

This wide interpatient variability seen with a subdural block may be explained by its anatomical basis. Ultrastructural studies have demonstrated that there is no space between the dura and the arachnoid but the so-called subdural space is not a potential space as previously thought, but is only produced as a result of trauma and tissue damage creating a cleft within the meninges [22] (Fig. 2.19).

The arachnoid mater has an outer compact laminar portion attached to the inside of the dural sac and a separate inner trabeculated portion. Between the laminar arachnoid portion and the dura there is a compartment termed the dura-arachnoid interface. This dura-arachnoid interface is composed of neurothelial cells having relatively few intercellular joints and large intercellular lacunae filled with an amorphous material. This suggests that iatrogenic dissection of this cellular plane can occur if neurothelial cells break up on application of pressure by mechanical forces such as air or fluid injection (Fig. 9.3). Thus fissures can be created within the dura-arachnoid interface, with considerable variability in form. While some fissures remain incomplete, some expand towards weaker areas creating a subdural space. These fissures may combine to form the so-called primary subdural space which may be short or may, sometimes, extend to almost the whole length of the vertebral column and occasionally into the cranial cavity. Injection of a sufficient amount of local anesthetic into this primary subdural space may result in sign and symptoms of an extensive block, with apnea and unconsciousness in the most severe cases. Parallel to this primary space a number of secondary subdural spaces encroaching into the dura may also create the so-called intradural space which is radiologically distinguishable from the "subdural space." Also the intradural space is artifactual and is formed by dural delamination produced by needle or catheter insertion into the dural lamina thickness (Fig. 9.4).

The mechanism underlying intradural catheter placement may be considered as a "tenting effect" during advancement of the epidural needle once the dura is reached. If enough pressure is exerted, the tip of the needle may partially pierce some of the dural layers, allowing the passage of the catheter between these layers, creating an intradural space. Injection of air, saline, contrast, or other solutions would encourage laminar detachment, thus expanding this space within the thickness of the dura [23].

9.2.2   Subdural Block

A subdural block can have a variable presentation depending upon the extent of the spread of local anesthetic, which in turn is dictated by the highly variable anatomical features of the created space itself. The onset of the block is somewhat intermediate between that of a subarachnoid and epidural block. The block is thus often characterized by a slow onset (approximately 15–20 min after drug injection) and usually lasts for up to 2 h, followed by a full recovery. The sensory block produced by subdural injection is usually high and disproportionate to the volume of drug injected, as the

Fig. 9.3 Subdural placement of an epidural catheter (scanning electron microscopy ×25) (from Reina et al. (2015) Atlas of functional anatomy for regional anesthesia and pain medicine. Springer, with permission)

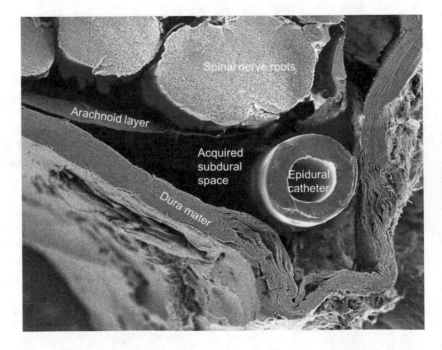

Fig. 9.4 Scanning electron microscopy image of an epidural catheter within the intradural space (scanning electron microcopy ×25 (**a**) and ×20 (**b**)) (from Reina et al. (2015) Atlas of functional anatomy for regional anesthesia and pain medicine. Springer, with permission, and from [23] with permission)

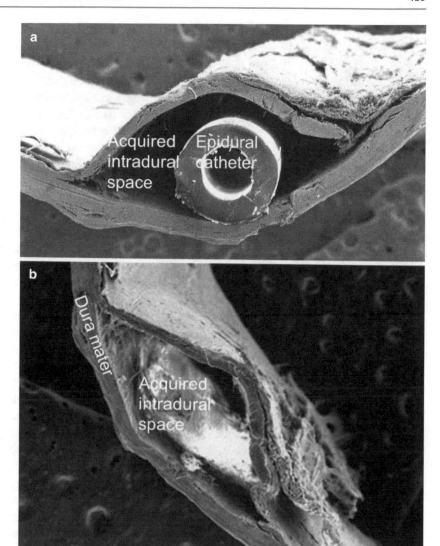

limited capacity of the space results in extensive spread. On the other hand, the sensory block may be inadequate or completely absent. There is usually sparing of or minimal effect on sympathetic and motor functions due to the relative sparing of the ventral nerve roots. Thus, hypotension is likely to be only moderate. Development of motor weakness is slow and less profound, with, in the most severe cases, progressive respiratory incoordination rather than sudden apnea.

However, unusual presentations of subdural block are not uncommon: significant motor weakness in the intercostal muscles and upper extremities, a faster rather than a slower onset of block, delayed onset, significant hypotension, and unilat-

eral block. In addition, because the subdural space extends intracranially unconsciousness and apnea may be produced which may last several hours.

Rarely, permanent neural damage can occur as a result of the compression of nerve roots or the radicular arteries traversing the space, causing ischemia of neural tissues [24].

9.2.3 Intradural Block

Whereas accidental injection of local anesthetic into the subdural space may produce an extensive block that may occasionally be life threatening, local anesthetic injected into the intradural space

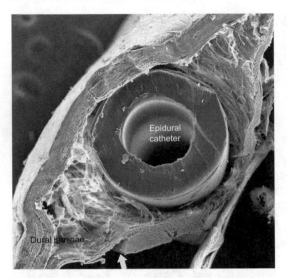

Fig. 9.5 Scanning electron microscopy image of an epidural catheter within the intradural space. The arrow indicates an area of breakage of dural laminae, caused by the catheter migrating towards the subarachnoid space (scanning electron microcopy ×50) (from Reina et al. (2015) Atlas of functional anatomy for regional anesthesia and pain medicine. Springer, with permission, and from [23] with permission)

appears to form a localized and swelling collection within the distal layers of the dura, producing a restricted, inadequate neuraxial block. Sometimes patients with an intradural block may develop pain during the epidural catheter insertion or with the injection of the anesthetic solution. This pain may be explained by the anterior swelling of the intradural mass coming into contact with the nerve roots.

Repeated doses of local anesthetic may escape from the intradural space, most likely around the outside of the epidural catheter, and eventually produce a clinically acceptable block. However, at least in theory, the anesthetic solution may also escape from the intradural space to the subdural space, following the rupture of the enclosing layers of dura or to the subarachnoid space, following the rupture of the surrounding dura and arachnoid (Fig. 9.5).

9.3   Neurologic Injuries After Epidural Block

The majority of neurologic injuries are not directly attributable to anesthetic interventions but rather are intrinsic to labor and delivery or

may even occur spontaneously. Neuraxial complications from anesthetic techniques include direct trauma due to pressure exerted by a needle or catheter on spinal nerve roots, epidural hematoma, and epidural abscess. Fortunately, these are very rare but they can be neurologically devastating if unrecognized. In the obstetric population the calculated incidence of neurologic injuries after an epidural block is 1/25,000 [25] and the incidence of permanent nerve damage is between 0.2 and 1.2/100,000 [26] or 4 per million [27].

With all neuraxial complications, the longer it takes to diagnose and treat, the worse the prognosis is. Infections such as epidural abscess and meningitis are very rare and may be a manifestation of systemic sepsis. Epidural hematoma usually occurs in association with coagulation defects; however, it may also occur spontaneously, unrelated to epidural block.

Most neurologic complications following childbirth are intrinsic obstetric palsies which may be more, as frequent as 0.9% of deliveries [28].

Peripheral nerve injury after labor and delivery may result from operative delivery, lithotomy position, or compression by the fetal head and may occur even in the absence of neuraxial technique. In the past obstetric practice allowed protracted labor and frequent use of forceps, which contributed to lumbosacral plexus injury. The fetal head may also compress and injure the lumbosacral plexus as it crosses the ala of the sacrum or the posterior brim of the pelvis. This injury is more common in nulliparous women with platypelloid pelvis, large babies, cephalopelvic disproportion, vertex presentation, and forceps delivery. Compressive nerve injuries of this type may involve multiple root levels and appear as injuries to the femoral or obturator nerves with sensory impairment in the fourth and fifth lumbar dermatomes. Femoral nerve injury decreases sensation over the anterior thigh and medial calf and impairs quadriceps strength, hip flexion, and patellar reflex. Proximal lesions at the level of the lumbosacral plexus may also decrease hip flexion due to iliopsoas weakness. The obturator nerve can be compressed against the lateral pelvic wall or during its course in the obturator canal. This results in decreased sensation over the medial thigh, weakness of the hip adductors, and decreased ability to internally rotate.

9.3.1 Needle/Catheter Trauma

Single-root neuropathies due to direct trauma to the nerve root with an epidural needle are very rare (0.75/10,000) [29].

A combination of intraneural intrafascicular needle placement and high injection pressures may lead to severe fascicular injury and persistent neurologic deficits [30].

Transient paresthesias are not uncommon when threading an epidural catheter and are unlikely to cause nerve damage.

However, painful or persistent paresthesias are much more concerning for nerve injury. The needle or catheter must be removed or repositioned immediately and the patient followed closely postpartum. Likewise, any paresthesia or pain elicited by injection of local anesthetic down a needle or catheter should result in cessation of injection and close follow-up. Two-thirds of anesthesia-related neurological complications are associated with either paresthesia (direct nerve trauma) or pain during injection (intraneuronal location) [31].

Paresthesia, loss of sensation, and muscular weakness in the distribution of the nerve are commonly observed.

Flexible catheters are less traumatizing than the more rigid variety, but can still wrap around nerve roots or become stuck in intervertebral foramina. Damage to the underlying spinal cord can occur, either as a consequence of incautious advancement of the epidural needle or as secondary to abnormal anatomy, such as a tethered cord in patients with spina bifida.

All paresthesias should be documented and followed up postpartum. The absence of any paresthesia or pain during a neuraxial procedure makes any nerve injury much more likely to be obstetric in origin; in addition most obstetric neuropathies are not painful, and symptoms are either unchanged or improving by the time patients complain of them. Neuropathies related to neuraxial anesthesia are frequently painful

with worsening symptoms. Severe back pain and generalized lower extremity numbness and weakness with or without sphincter dysfunction are highly suggestive of a central lesion compromising the spinal cord.

Most intrinsic obstetric peripheral nerve injuries are temporary and will spontaneously resolve within 6–8 weeks. Some may take longer. Treatment is supportive with physical therapy playing a major role to avoid muscle atrophy.

Recovery of nerve injury secondary to neuraxial procedures depends on the site and severity of the injury. Mild injuries will resolve in a similar time course to obstetric neuropathies, but severe injuries may have complete or partial loss of function.

9.3.2 Epidural Hematoma

Epidural hematoma is a feared, but rarely seen, complication of regional anesthesia in 1 in 168,000 women, or 6 per million [27].

Most epidural hematomas following regional anesthesia occur in patients with hemostatic abnormalities, particularly those on anticoagulants or in patients with severe preeclampsia [32–34].

The symptoms of epidural hematoma are bilateral leg weakness, urinary incontinence, and loss of rectal sphincter tone. These severe neurologic deficits may be preceded by sharp pain in the back or legs with progression over a few hours. Prolonged motor paralysis without regression of block should raise suspicion. Symptomatic epidural hematoma must be decompressed surgically within 6 h for the best chance of a full recovery.

Spontaneous epidural hematoma may occur very rarely in pregnancy. Pregnancy is characterized by a relatively hypercoagulable state, effectively reducing the risk of epidural hematoma. However, the epidural space houses an extensive venous system containing tributaries from the spinal cord and vertebral bodies that drain into the external vertebral venous plexus and become more engorged during pregnancy. Because this venous system does not contain valves, and exists within a low-pressure environment, any pressure exerted proximally because of a Valsalva maneuver, vomiting, or mechanical compression of the vena cava can dramatically increase the transmural venous pressure, leaving the veins vulnerable to injury. It has been postulated that spontaneous epidural hematoma may occur from preexisting faults in the venous wall exacerbated by well-described mechanical and hyperdynamic conditions existing in the peripartum period [35].

9.3.3 Epidural Abscess

Only 3.9% of all epidural abscesses are associated with anesthetic interventions [36] and, in addition, they are even more infrequent among obstetric patients [37].

This is not surprising, since the major risk factors for epidural abscess are compromised immunity, disruption of spinal column, and long-term epidural catheterization, all factors rarely occurring in pregnant women.

Symptoms include fever, malaise, headache, and back pain at the level of the infection. There may be evidence of superficial infection at the needle/catheter insertion site, and pain is found on deep palpation over the site. The white blood cell count is elevated. Progression of symptoms to nerve root pain usually takes 1–3 days. Neurologic deficits will progress as the spinal cord is compressed including lower extremity pain, weakness, bowel and bladder dysfunction, and paraplegia. Surgical treatment is necessary.

9.4 Epidural Catheter Breakage

Epidural catheter breakage is very rare and anecdotic and, except for a few instances, is a benign issue.

Actions that may favor the breakage of an epidural catheter during its insertion may be inserting an excessive length of the catheter; exerting excessive force to advance the catheter against resistance; withdrawing the catheter without at the same time withdrawing the Tuohy needle; and advancing the Tuohy needle over the cath-

eter. In addition the catheter may be damaged if pinched between the tip of the needle and a bony surface. In theory, when CSE is performed at different interspaces, the catheter may get sheared off the by spinal needle.

Most frequently the breakage of the catheter occurs during its removal especially if excessive force is applied to remove a knotted, kinked, or entrapped catheter or when the catheter has taken a circuitous course around any tissue such as bone, fascia, ligament, or nerve and an excessive pulling force is applied. Catheters may also get broken due to manufacturing defect.

Suggested maneuvers to prevent epidural catheter fracture during its insertion are the following: excessive insertion should be avoided to prevent coiling, knotting, and entrapment of the catheter [38, 39].

On encountering resistance, the catheter should never be withdrawn through the needle and both the needle and the catheter should be removed as a single unit. A catheter should be checked for manufacturing defects and a sharp bevel tip should be ruled out.

Suggested maneuvers to prevent epidural catheter fracture during its removal are the following: if resistance or stretching of the catheter occurs while attempting withdrawal, it is recommended to place patients in the same position as they were at the time of insertion [40]. A flexed lateral decubitus position is reported to be more effective than the sitting position, with withdrawal forces being as much as 2.5 times greater in the sitting position [41].

In the case of a difficult catheter removal the efforts at removal should be discontinued for 15–30 min allowing tissue relaxation [40]. Injection of saline solution through the catheter with simultaneous slow but firm traction can also be performed [42].

In a difficult removal situation, one can choose between incision under local anesthesia with sedation and general anesthesia with muscle relaxants.

All patients with a retained epidural catheter fragment should undergo proper imaging studies to know its exact location. It is also necessary for documentation purposes and to encourage asymptomatic patients to have a timely follow-up so that an earliest possible diagnosis of symptoms can be made. Radiographies, computed tomography, magnetic resonance imaging, and ultrasonography have all been used with variable results.

Surgical removal is indicated only in complicated cases such as leaking CSF through the catheter whose tip is either placed or has migrated to the intrathecal space and is now acting as a wick, or when either the patient develops infection or radicular pain due to nerve entrapment, or when the broken end of the catheter is emerging out of the skin, acting as a portal of entry for infection.

References

1. Choi PT, Lucas S. Postdural puncture headache. In: Halpern SH, Douglas MJ, editors. Evidence-based obstetric anesthesia. Malden: Blackwell Publishing; 2005. p. 192–207.
2. Webb CA, Weyker PD, Zhang L, et al. Unintentional dural puncture with a Tuohy needle increases risk of chronic headache. Anesth Analg. 2012;115:124–32.
3. Reina MA, López-García A, de Andrés-Ibáñez JA, et al. Electron microscopy of the lesions produced in the human dura mater by Quincke beveled and Whitacre needles. Rev Esp Anestesiol Reanim. 1997;44:56–61.
4. Reina MA, López A, van Zundert A, et al. Ultrastructure of dural lesions produced in lumbar punctures. In: Reina MA, editor. Atlas of functional anatomy of regional anesthesia and pain medicine. New York: Springer; 2015. p. 767–94.
5. Reina MA, Castedo J, López A. Postdural puncture headache. Ultrastructure of dural lesions and spinal needles used in lumbar punctures. Rev Arg Anestesiol. 2008;66:6–26.
6. Reina MA, Prats-Galino A, Sola RG, et al. Structure of the arachnoid layer of the human spinal meninges: a barrier that regulates dural sac permeability. Rev Esp Anestesiol Reanim. 2010;57(8):486–92.
7. Reina MA, López A, Badorrey V, et al. Dura-arachnoid lesions produced by 22 gauge Quincke spinal needles during a lumbar puncture. J Neurol Neurosurg Psychiatry. 2004;75:893–7.
8. Lybecker H, Djernes M, Schmidt JF. Postdural puncture headache (PDPH): onset, duration, severity, and associated symptoms. An analysis of 75 consecutive patients with PDPH. Acta Anaesthesiol Scand. 1995;39:605–12.
9. HIS classification. https://ichd-3.org/7-headache-attributed-to-non-vascular-intracranial-disorder/7-2-headache-attributed-to-low-cerebrospinal-fluid-pressure/7-2-1-post-dural-puncture-headache/.
10. Angle P, Thompson D, Halpern S, et al. Second stage pushing correlates with headache after unintentional dural puncture in parturients. Can J Anaesth. 1999;46:861–6.
11. Sadashivaiah J, McLure H. 18-G Tuohy needle can reduce the incidence of severe post dural puncture headache. Anaesthesia. 2009;64:1379–80.
12. De Almeida SM, Shumaker SD, LeBlanc SK, et al. Incidence of postdural puncture headache in research volunteers. Headache. 2011;51:1503–10.
13. Arevalo-RodriguezI,CiapponiA,MunozL,etal.Posture and fluids for preventing post-dural puncture headache. Cochrane Database Syst Rev. 2013;(7):CD009199. https://doi.org/10.1002/14651858.CD009199.pub2.
14. Apfel CC, Saxena OS, Cakmakkaya OS, et al. Prevention of postdural puncture headache after accidental dural puncture: a quantitative systematic review. Br J Anaesth. 2010;105:255–63.
15. Heesen M, Klohr S, Rossaint R, et al. Can incidence of accidental dural puncture in laboring women be reduced? A systematic review and meta analysis. Minerva Anestesiol. 2013;79:1187–97.
16. Reina M, Lirk P, Sàncez AP, et al. Human lumbar ligamentum flavum anatomy for epidural anesthesia. Reviewing a 3D MR-based interactive model and postmortem samples. Anesth Analg. 2016;122:903–7.
17. Russcl R, Laxton C, Lucas DN, et al. Treatment of obstetric postdural puncture headache. Part 1: conservative and pharmacological management. Int J Obstet Anesth. 2019;38:93–103.
18. Russell R, Laxton C, Lucas DN, et al. Treatment of obstetric post dural puncture headache. Part 2: epidural blood patch. Int J Obstet Anesth. 2019;38:104–18.
19. Paech MJ, Doherty DA, Christmas T, et al. The volume of blood for epidural blood patch in obstetrics: a randomized blinded clinical trial. Anesth Analg. 2011;113:126–33.
20. Lubenow T, Keh-Wong E, Kristof K, et al. Inadvertent subdural injection: a complication of an epidural block. Anesth Analg. 1988;67:175–9.
21. Jenkins JG. Some immediate serious complications of obstetric epidural analgesia and anaesthesia: a prospective study of 145,550 epidurals. Int J Obstet Anesth. 2005;14:37–42.
22. Reina MA, De Leon CO, Lòpez A, et al. The origin of the spinal subdural space: ultrastructure findings. Anesth Analg. 2002;94:991–5.
23. Collier CB, Reina MA, Prats-Galino A, et al. An anatomical study of the intradural space. Anaesth Intensive Care. 2011;39:1038–42.
24. Mc Menemin IM, Sissons GR, Brownridge P. Accidental subdural catheterization: radiological evidence of a possible mechanism for spinal cord damage. Br J Anaesth. 1992;69:417–9.
25. Moen V, Dahlgren N, Irestedt L. Severe neurological complications after central neuraxial blockades in Sweden 1990–1999. Anesthesiology. 2004;10:950–9.
26. Royal College of Anaesthetists. 3rd National Audit Project (NAP3). National Audit of Major

Complications of Central Neuraxial Block in the United Kingdom; 2009.

27. Ruppen W, Derry S, McQuay H, et al. Incidence of epidural hematoma, infection and neurologic injury in obstetric patients with epidural analgesia/anesthesia. Anesthesiology. 2006;105:394–9.

28. Wong CA, Scavone BM, Dugan S, et al. Incidence of postpartum lumbosacral spine and lower extremity nerve injuries. Obstet Gynecol. 2003;101:279–88.

29. Scott DB, Tunstall ME. Serious complications associated with epidural/spinal blockade in obstetrics: a two-year prospective study. Int J Obstet Anesth. 1995;4:133–9.

30. Gentili F, Hudson AR, Hunter D, et al. Nerve injection injury with local anesthetic agents: a light and electron microscopic, fluorescent microscopic, and horseradish peroxidase study. Neurosurgery. 1980;6:263–72.

31. Auroy Y, Narchi P, Messiah A, et al. Serious complications related to regional anesthesia: results of a prospective survey in France. Anesthesiology. 1997;87:479–86.

32. Horlocker TT. Regional anesthesia and analgesia in the patient receiving thromboprophylaxis. [editorial]. Reg Anesth. 1996;21:503–7.

33. Lao TT, Halpern SH, MacDonald D, et al. Spinal subdural haematoma in a parturient after attempted epidural anaesthesia. Can J Anaesth. 1993;40:340–5.

34. Yuen TS, Kua JSW, Tan IKS. Spinal haematoma following epidural anaesthesia in a patient with eclampsia. Anaesthesia. 2002;50:350–71.

35. Carroll SG. Spontaneous spinal extradural hematoma during pregnancy. J Matern Fetal Med. 1997;6:218–9.

36. Reihsaus E, Waldbaur H, Seeling W. Spinal epidural abscess: a meta-analysis of 915 patients. Neurosurg Rev. 2000;23:175–204.

37. Loo CC, Dahlgren G, Irestedt L. Neurological complications in obstetric regional anaesthesia. Int J Obstet Anesth. 2000;9:99–124.

38. Schummer W, Schummer C. Another cause of epidural catheter breakage? Anesth Analg. 2002;94:233.

39. Hobaika AB. Breakage of epidural catheters: etiology, prevention, and management. Rev Bras Anestesiol. 2008;58:227–33.

40. Morris GN, Warren BB, Hanson EW, et al. Influence of patient position on withdrawal forces during removal of lumbar extradural catheters. Br J Anaesth. 1996;77:419–20.

41. Demiraran Y, Yucel I, Erdogmus B. Subcutaneous effusion resulting from an epidural catheter fragment. Br J Anaesth. 2006;96:508–9.

42. Podovei M, Flaherty D, San Vicente M, et al. Epidural saline to facilitate arrow flex-tip epidural catheter removal. Anesth Analg. 2011;112:1251.

Teaching the Epidural Block

Epidural block is a complex procedure and requires cognitive skills such as the knowledge of the anatomy and of the procedure along with psychomotor skills such as the skills required to perform the technique.

In the past, the beginner typically prepared himself/herself by appropriate introductory reading and then apprentice and master approached the task together in the clinical setting, with live patients as the learning model. Inevitably this model determined a certain number of inadvertent dural punctures which had to be accepted as part of a necessary teaching system committed to develop the future care of patients.

In some hospitals novice anesthesiologists still undergo training directly on patients, while in others they can use simulation and simulators before going to the patient.

10.1 Teaching the Epidural Block

An ideal sequence to be used during the training might be as follows: firstly the residents undertake basic formal training to gain knowledge and skills including lectures, video, and audiovisual aids and practice the procedure on simulators; secondly the residents may observe the experts carrying out the procedure on the patient and thereafter perform the procedure under the supervision of the experienced anesthesiologist; and finally they perform the procedure alone. Direct observation, checklists, rating scales, and learning curves may eventually be used to determine whether the trainee has reached the adequate level of competence. Videotaping and video review of trainees may also help in acquiring epidural skills and it is a promising, valuable tool in training and motivating anesthesiology residents initiating epidural analgesia on the labor and delivery ward [1].

In practice, there is no universally accepted, comprehensive, or standard systematic way to teach the epidural block.

However, undoubtedly the transition from a situation where trainees are taught epidural block on patients directly and deemed competent mainly on the discretion of a supervising anesthesiologist to a more structured epidural training program which also includes simulation and a designed supervising and teaching model may improve the teaching and greatly decrease the accidental dural puncture rate during the period of training [2].

There are three stages in the acquisition of procedural skills: cognition, integration, and automation. Cognition includes developing an understanding of the task, and perceptual awareness. It is assisted by a clear description and demonstrations of the task. In the integration stage, the knowledge from the cognition phase is incorporated into the learning of the motor skills for that task. Ultimately, the task becomes automatic and even subconscious. For an expert, and thus

G. Capogna, *Epidural Technique In Obstetric Anesthesia*,
https://doi.org/10.1007/978-3-030-45332-9_10

for a teacher, it may not be easy to break a task down into component parts in order to teach a novice. It may also be hard to understand what the most frequent difficult steps are for a novice to overcome.

The major basic difficulties encountered by beginners in the epidural procedure include:

(a) The ability to identify the interspace and give the needle the orientation at the desired angle so that no bone contacts result

(b) The ability to identify false or pseudo losses of resistance: In some institutions, when the epidural block is taught the needle is introduced a few centimeters into the soft tissues and not to the dorsal aspect of the ligamentum flavum because of the fear of puncturing the dura and in order to make the trainee more comfortable. In this way the needle may be located somewhere between the soft tissues, well before the epidural space, and if the LORT with syringe procedure is initiated at this stage it may give rise to a false loss of resistance.

(c) The ability to recognize bone contact and correctly redirect the needle on the right path in accordance with the angle of inclination of the needle, its depth, the position of the vertebrae, and the tactile sensations returned by the needle itself.

(d) The ability to place the needle in the epidural space with a reasonable extension without puncturing the dura: Extension is defined as the distance the needle tip goes beyond the ligamentum flavum into the epidural space: the less the overshoot the less likely the dural puncture will be. The extension of the needle depends on various factors, such as human perception, tissue parameters (peak force in ligamentum flavum, the drop force), and human factors such as the hand position holding the needle, muscle co-contraction (making the wrist and finger joints of both hands stiff), and needle velocity. Experts are able to control the extension by regulating the pressure exerted on the needle-syringe-piston system, controlling needle velocity,

and perceiving the force changes while novices do not have this ability.

10.2 Teaching Tools

10.2.1 Epidural Simulators

Manikin epidural simulators are task trainers based upon physical manikin or dummy models made from plastic or rubber. They are not computer driven and generally contain no mechanical or electronic parts or technology. They are portable, easy to set up and use, and may have physically palpable anatomical landmarks. Several simulators based on plastic human-shaped models have been developed. These often contain solid structures to represent the lumbar vertebrae. The surface is covered with an artificial synthetic skin, which is often replaceable with various densities to represent patient variation. There is often a composite rubber spinal canal, filled with a liquid to mimic CSF. If punctured with a needle, CSF leak occurs in vivo. A few manikin simulators are amenable to ultrasound (US) scanning allowing the internal structures to be viewed prepuncture and an estimate made as to the depth and location of the epidural space.

Manikin simulators have the advantage of looking similar to a patient. They are easy to setup, portable, and usually cheaper. The main advantage is that manikins are physical rather than virtual, and since a clinician uses his/her hands to perform the epidural insertion a physical simulator may be a closer analogy. For example, the manikins often contain a saline-filled dural sac which can leak if the dura is punctured and the operator can remove the skin and look inside at the physical parts, which helps to envisage the spinal anatomy. One disadvantage of manikin simulators is that the accuracy of tissues is hard to reproduce with artificial rubber or plastics. The majority of insertion forces have been designed using the opinions of expert clinicians trying an insertion and giving feedback, but they are not based on actual recorded data. Moreover, it is difficult for manikins to contain and reproduce all of the precise anatomical layers such as skin, subcutaneous fat, various ligaments, meningeal layers, and bone.

Recent developments in the area of haptics and virtual reality technologies have led to the development of virtual reality-based epidural simulators with haptic feedback.

Haptic technology can better mimic the forces needed to cross the tissues during the epidural block and real-time 3D visualization allows the needle to be seen from all angles and its location in relation to internal spinal anatomy.

Commercially available simulators are very expensive and still have some limitations associated with the use of a commercially available haptic device, such as reduced needle insertion mobility, limited force range, and performance in orienting the needle.

New and more sophisticated types of simulators are currently in their early stages of development (prototype level). Realistic simulation is possible, the trainee's task can be recorded, and varying patient anatomy can be simulated. In these simulators, the computer displays a 3D patient model with a vertebral column and a polygon model of the needle. The 3D patient model data came from magnetic resonance image (MRI) scans of actual patients. Haptic forces are based on data obtained during epidural insertions from a variety of tissues including canine, porcine, and postmortem human and live human volunteers, combined with expert opinion. This force data describes the forces encountered on the Tuohy needle as it is inserted.

Software and haptics replicate the conditions of giving an epidural to a real-life patient, allowing adjustments for different heights, BMIs, angles, and rotations of the spine [3].

The virtual patient can adjust to various body shapes, sizes, weights, and heights. Since body size considerably affects the insertion force, the haptic device can recreate forces for each body size. The spine in this 3D model can bend and flex in real time, to allow simulation of various patient positions including sitting, lying on the side, lateral decubitus, and flexing, which increases the spacing between vertebrae. A 3D immersive monitor is incorporated with reflective polarized images allowing for 3D visualization of the complete procedure from various viewing angles.

In the future for obstetric anesthesia training mannequins with anatomy similar to a parturient are needed, which can simulate the movements of women during labor contractions. Such a mannequin (for obstetric anesthesia simulation training) would ideally also need to be kept in an environment where the sound of the cardiotocography is audible, and the setting is as stressful as a delivery room with paramedical staff and attendants. Robotic mannequins with artificial intelligence or, better, hybrid simulators with human actors could be the next-generation tools for obstetric anesthesia training.

10.2.2 Continuous Real-Time Pressure-Sensing Technology

The Dynamic Pressure Sensing® (DPS) technology (CompuFlo Epidural Trainer®) (see Chap. 6) (Fig. 10.1) can differentiate tissue types by pressure signatures that are imperceptible to touch. This allows the trainee to accurately identify the needle location and discriminate between false and true loss of resistance. By connecting tactile feel with real-time and objective visual and audible confirmation of all pressure changes, trainees can verify that they have accessed the ligamentum flavum and/or the epidural space, building confidence and speeding the procedure's learning curve. The instrument may be used with patients [4] and with epidural simulators as well [5, 6].

An additional novel and an important feature of this instrument is that it allows to have a documented data set and graph correlating to the performing procedure and this enables trainers/trainees to review the procedure after it is completed and critique the procedure. Documentation of a technique and/or procedure can lead to best practices of a technique and allows for objective research to be conducted as well. Having displayed, recorded, and printed a graph illustrating the procedure may also lead to a greater appreciation of the anatomy and the structures an operator must contend with thus lead to a more rapid mastery of the technique.

Fig. 10.1 The CompuFlo Epidural Trainer® uses the Dynamic Pressure Sensing® (DPS) technology and allows the trainee to accurately identify the epidural needle location

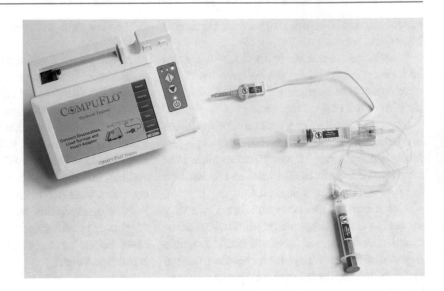

10.3 Learning Assessment

Direct observation by an expert instructor is traditionally used to assess procedural skills and this is nicely feasible in anesthesia because of the high degree of supervision in cases performed by trainees. Despite being feasible, assessments without specific criteria result in poor reliability and validity. Determining the point at which a trainee is deemed capable of working independently on the labor ward is challenging, and a robust method of evaluating competence would be highly desirable.

10.3.1 Direct Observation with Checklists and Rating Scales

To overcome these problems, direct observation with specific criteria has been developed.

Structured direct observation of procedural skills (DOPS) is a method designed to provide feedback on procedural skills essential to the provision of good clinical care.

The assessment involves an assessor observing the trainee perform a practical procedure within the workplace and a structured checklist is designed to give guidance for the assessors.

Binary content checklists can be used as a way of grading performance during direct observation. Checklists break a task down into its component parts and assign a dichotomous pass/fail outcome to each point. A new checklist needs to be designed and validated for each procedural skill that is to be assessed. Checklists can be constructed by surveying experts, although a different group of experts may not agree on each point of the checklist. Checklists have been found to have excellent reliability in the assessment of epidural anesthesia even if published checklists for epidural anesthesia may greatly differ between them, having so many different items on their lists [7–10] (Fig. 10.2).

Checklists have also been designed with outcomes of "not performed," "performed poorly," and "performed well" rather than a binary pass/fail outcome to allow them to become more qualitative at the cost of a loss in objectivity. A potential problem with checklists is that if all stages are weighted equally regardless of clinical importance, then a trainee may be able to obtain a high score, despite omitting important stages.

Global rating scales (GRSs) [7] (Fig. 10.3) differ from checklists, in that they use a Likert scale rather than a dichotomous outcome. As the GRS has a gradation of response in each category, it is less objective than a checklist, although

Fig. 10.2 Task-specific checklist for epidural anesthesia (adapted from [7] with permission)

✅ CHECKLIST for EPIDURAL ANESTHESIA

1. Ensures patient is positioned comfortably and safely in the middle of the bed
2. Adjusts height of bed appropriately
3. Carefully prepares a sterile work surface
4. Pours antiseptic solution (or has nurse pour it) without contaminating the epidural set
5. Washes hands and puts on gloves in a sterile fashion
6. Optimally positions him/herself for the procedure
7. Prepares the skin at the back widely and aseptically
8. Allows solution to dry
9. Neatly lays out and prepares all necessary equipment (needles, syringes, local anesthetic)
10. Asks patient to arch her back
11. Places drape over patient's back in a sterile fashion
12. Landmarks site of injection after palpating iliac crests
13. Warns patient of needle insertion
14. Infiltrates subcutaneous layers with local anesthetic
15. Places epidural needle with correct positioning of bevel
16. Inserts epidural needle through skin, subcutaneous tissue, and into ligament before attaching the syringe
17. Attaches air/saline filled syringe to the needle hub with needle well controlled
18. Braces hand/s holding the needle against patient's back in complete control of the needle
19. Slowly advances needle through supraspinous and interspinous ligaments and into ligamentum flavum while applying pressure on the plunger (continuous or intermittent)
20. Identifies LOR and immediately releases pressure on the plunger
21. Notes depth of needle insertion before threading catheter
22. Warns patient about possible paresthesia during catheter threading
23. Detaches the syringe and threads the catheter to a depth of 4-5 cm
24. Pulls the needle out while maintaining correct catheter placement
25. Carefully aspirates from catheter
26. Injects test dose through flushed filter
27. Fixes the epidural catheter securely

this allows the assessment to be more qualitative. GRS can be used to assess many different skills and they are the most objective way that aspects of performance such as professionalism and interpersonal skills can be assessed. When used to assess procedural skill, either a GRS may describe an overall impression of the quality of performance or there may be a Likert scale for a number of different domains within an overall performance. GRS can be used prospectively or retrospectively, although, as in other forms of assessment, there is evidence that reliability is poor if used retrospectively. Potential pitfalls with GRS include the "halo effect," when good or bad performance in one domain unduly influences the grading of performance in other domains.

	1	2	3	4	5
Preparation for procedure	Did not organize equipment well. Has to stop procedure frequently to prepare equipment		Equipment generally organized. Occasionally has to stop and prepare items.		All equipment neatly organized, prepared and ready for use
Respect for tissue	Frequently used unnecessary force on tissue or caused damage		Careful handing of tissue but occasionally caused indadvertent damage		Consistently handled tissues appropriately with minimal damage
Time and motion	Many unnecessary moves		Efficient time/motion but some unnecessary moves		Clear economy of movement and maximum efficiency
Instrument handling	Repeated makes tentative or awkward moves with instruments		Competent use of instruments but occasionally appeared stiff or awkward		Fluid moves with instruments and no awkwardness
Flow of procedure	Frequently stopped procedure and seemed unsure of next move		Demontrated some forward planning with resonable progression of procedure		Obviously planned course of procedure with effortless flow from one move to the next
Knowledge of procedure	Deficient knowledge		Knew all important steps of procedure		Demonstrated familiarity with all aspects of procedure
Overall performance	Very poor		Competent		Clearly superior

Fig. 10.3 The Global Rating Scale (GRS) (adapted from [7] with permission)

The main advantages of the structured direct observation of procedural skills as an assessment tool are the following: (a) the trainee is assessed performing procedures on real patients during everyday work; (b) not only the technical ability is observed, but also interaction with patients, colleagues, and professional behavior can be assessed; (c) a wide range of skills, from simple to very complex procedures, can be assessed; (d) many trainees will "need further development," so after receiving feedback, the strengths and weaknesses can be highlighted and the trainee can work on them and be assessed at a later date.

Another additional method for evaluating trainees is videotaping and video reviewing which may result in greater improvement in overall and selected performance criteria. With this method, one or more independent observers may review the videos by using previously established criteria [1] (Fig. 10.4).

10.3.2 Learning Curves

In 1936, Wright, an aeronautical engineer, published the first description of a learning curve [11]. He hypothesized that speed or efficiency of airplane component production increased, and costs decreased, as the experience and skill of the workforce increased. In industry measures of performance are often obvious, but in medicine it is more difficult to assess a clinicians' performance. Measures of learning related to a medical (anesthetic) technique fall into two categories: measures of anesthetic process and measures of patient outcome. Process outcomes are generally easier to analyze and therefore more commonly used, though they are only indirectly related to patient outcomes.

The need for appropriate indices of outcomes has been recognized and multidimensional plots taking into account all significant variables are most likely to give the most accurate representation of a specific operation's learning curve.

A hypothetical plot is illustrated in Fig. 10.5 which has four main phases. The starting coordinate A represents start of training. Secondly, the curve ascends. The gradient of this ascent indicates how quickly the individuals' performance improves; this part of the curve may be a stepwise ascent as individuals learn and master stages of a complex procedure. Improvements in performance tend to be most rapid at first and then tail off, as the degree of improvement

CRITERIA FOR ASSESSING TRAINEE'S COMPETENCE

Proper positioning

| Was the patient seated evenly (i.e., not on an angle) on the bed?
| Was the patient asked to "round" her back?
| Was the resident's position optimal for placement of the epidural?
| Was the bed height appropriate?
| After completion of the epidural, was uterine displacement attained?

No spillage

| Was the providone iodine solution poured without contaminating
| the epidural kit?

Draping

| Was the drape placed without contaminating the block site, gloves,
| or epidural kit?

Midline location

| Was the needle placed at the correct interspace (i.e., below the L2-L3
| interspace) and in the midline position?

Air amount

| Was an excessive amount (5 ml) of air injected into the epidural needle?

Needle withdrawal

| Was the needle withdrawn carefully and steadily without displacing the catheter?
| If the catheter could not be threaded, was the needle and catheter withdrawn
| together?

Gentle treatment

| Was the patient told that the disinfectant solution was about to be applied?
| Was the patient told of the impending needle stick prior to administration
| of local anesthetic?
| Was local anesthetic administered in an appropriate manner?
| Was the patient informed of the possibility of paresthesia at the time of
| catheter insertion?
| After taping, was the patient placed in a comfortable, non-injurious position?

Adhering to aseptic technique

| Where gloves put on sterilely?
| Was the sterile field contaminated at any point?
| Was the kit opened aseptically?
| Was the patent's balc circumferentially prepared?
| Where three seperate sponge sticks applied?
| Was sterile technique maintained during catheter insertion and taping?

Povidone iodine

| Was povidone iodine solution allowed to dry?
| Was adequate time allowed between sponge stick applications?

Needle control

| Was the needle advanced carefully and steadily?

Cephalad direction

| Was the needle incorrectly inserted in a cauded direction?

Catheter insertion

| Was the catheter advanced carefully?
| Was the length of catheter approoriate (i.e., approximately 5 cm into the
| epidural space)?
| Was the catheter withdrawn to the proper length, if necessary?

Catheter securing

| Was the catheter taped appropriately?
| Did the resident avoid the patient's hair during taping?
| Was the catheter aspirated?
| Was the epidural catheter secured without kinking or dispalcement?

Fig. 10.4   Criteria to evaluate epidural anesthesia video-taped performance skills (adapted from [1] with permission)

Fig. 10.5   A hypothetical learning curve. (a) Start of training; (b) the procedure can be performed independently and competently; (c) additional experience improves outcomes by small amounts; (d) plateau is reached; (e) fall in the level of performance (advancing age, deterioration of manual dexterity, eyesight, memory, and cognition)

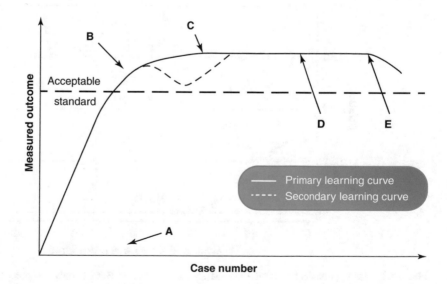

attained with each case reduces as the technique is refined. Thirdly, assuming adequate aptitude, a point is reached when the procedure can be performed independently and competently (coor-dinate B). Additional experience improves out-comes by small amounts (coordinate C), until a plateau, or asymptote, is reached (coordinate D). Fourthly, with advancing age, manual dexterity, eyesight, memory, and cognition may deteriorate, outweighing any advantage derived from long experience, leading to a fall in the level of performance (coordinate E). An alternative curve may also be drawn (dotted line), which exhibits temporary performance deterioration after technical competence has been achieved. The reasons postulated are case mix effect (undertaking more difficult cases), or overconfidence resulting in lapses in technique or judgement.

The learning curve is one of the most common tools to assess how the physician in training is progressing at a skill, and it is defined as a curve generated by plotting the success or failure against the number of attempts. With this method, approximately 20–25 procedures are necessary before improvement in the techniques of spinal and epidural anesthesia by residents in training, but if a 90% success rate is desired, 60 attempts at epidural anesthesia may be necessary [12].

More complex learning curves using an acceptable and unacceptable failure rate can be constructed. To perform these more complex learning curves a statistical tool such as the

cumulative sum technique (CUSUM) may be used [13] (Fig. 10.6). In this technique an acceptable and unacceptable failure rate is defined by discussion with experts. An acceptable success rate is defined, and the trainee gets a score for success or failure.

A CUSUM chart is basically a graphical representation of the trend in the outcomes of a series of consecutive procedures performed over time. It is designed to rapidly detect change in performance associated with an unacceptable rate of adverse outcome. At an acceptable level of performance, the CUSUM curve runs randomly at or above a horizontal line (no slope). However, when an individual is performing at an unacceptable level, the CUSUM curve slopes upward and will eventually cross a decision interval (horizontal lines drawn across a CUSUM chart), showing unsatisfactory performance. A skilled physician is expected to have a level CUSUM curve indicating ongoing maintenance of competence whereas a physician in training is expected to have a rising learning CUSUM curve. The degree of the slope is a measure of the progress in learn-

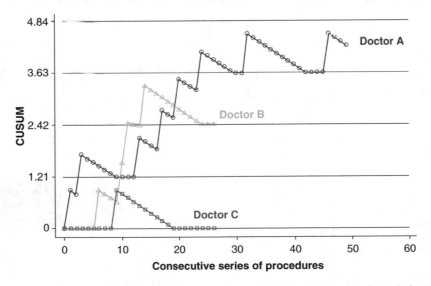

Fig. 10.6 The hypothetical upward CUSUM charts of three trainees, labeled as doctors A, B, and C. They performed 49, 26, and 26 procedures, respectively. The three trainees clearly demonstrated varying learning curves. Doctor C had no learning curve at all; his upward CUSUM curve was flat from the first procedure he attempted. Both doctor A and doctor B had a learning phase. However, doctor B took only 11 procedures before his upward CUSUM curve began to level, while doctor A required 23 procedures to achieve the same proficiency (adapted from Lim TO et al. (2002) Assessing Doctors' Competence: application of CUSUM technique in monitoring doctors' performance. Int J Quality Health Care 14: 251-258, with permission)

ing the new skill: the greater the slope, the slower the progress. When the curve eventually flattens (no slope), this indicates that the new skill has been learnt.

However, CUSUM analysis is a statistical method that investigates the outcome rather than the process of performing a procedural skill. The CUSUM chart allows the observer to decide whether a production process is in control (i.e., learning epidural technique) or it has become out of control, at which point the process needs to be halted, as the quality has decreased below acceptable limits. Using the CUSUM graphs the average number of obstetric epidurals needed to reach competence for inexperienced novices may greatly vary from 46 to 77, depending on the definition used for "success" [14].

The limitation of the learning curves is that the crude success rate ignores the context in which the epidurals were placed, such as, just to make some examples, the stage of labor, the anatomy of the patients, and the extent with which they were able to cooperate with attempts at their epidurals by novices. In addition, the success rate of trainees might be adversely affected if they were confronted with several difficult clinical situations in their first epidurals. Moreover, the successful placement of an epidural needle does not guarantee the successful placement of the epidural catheter nor its successful eventual management.

Learning curves provide only a snapshot of the trainee's performance. In the case of performance of a labor epidural, full competence is not necessarily achieved after a number of successful, directly observed attempts, but when the trainee is able to place and manage epidural labor analgesia consistently and successfully in multiple and different clinical situations.

10.3.3 Standardized Assessment After Simulation

Advances in simulation technology have enabled the evaluation of procedural skills to be taken out of the clinical context and into the simulation laboratory. This has created the possibility of standardized assessment of procedural skills.

Although simulation will never be exactly the same as a clinical experience, there are a number of advantages in assessing procedural skills in a simulated rather than in a clinical environment. Assessing procedural skills using a simulator answers to the ethical imperative to not harm patients. There is good evidence that simulation-based learning with task trainers, such as an epidural simulator, is effective for teaching procedural skills [15].

The haptic epidural simulator improves the performance of anesthesia trainees by reducing the number of bone contacts and the number of attempts, and by decreasing the procedure time [16].

However, even a simple model can be as useful for learning how to place an epidural catheter as an expensive anatomically correct simulator. A comparison between the efficacy of a high-fidelity epidural injection simulator (which includes a virtual reality display of the needle progression) with a "greengrocer's" model (inserting the epidural needle into a banana) showed no differences in trainees' epidural block performance on real patients [17].

In addition, it must be remembered that simulation is not only simulators. There is no difference between mental imagery and low-fidelity simulation training for epidural anesthesia skill acquisition. Both are capable of improvements in performance when allowed to practice and with the provision of immediate feedback. This supports the importance of effective scaffolding, a learning theory concept that describes the process of the basic support of a learner through interactions with an expert or another skilled peer, and the gradual adjustment and attenuation of this relationship as the learner progresses towards independence [18].

A reliable measure of technical skill is the "objective structured assessment of technical skills (OSATSs)" introduced to objectively assess procedural surgical skills outside the operating theatre [19]. Candidates perform a series of standardized surgical skills on bench models. At each time-limited station, candidates are examined by the direct observation of experts and technical skills are assessed using both a generic GRS and a task-specific checklist [20].

An OSATS examination format has not yet been used in anesthesia but simulation and multistation assessments similar to OSATS may become a key part of the future of procedural skill assessment in anesthesia if suitable part-task simulators can be validated. However, at the present time, there is not enough evidence to recommend that anesthesia trainees are evaluated in procedural skills using only simulators, especially when these skills can be reliably assessed by direct observation of performance on patients.

10.3.4 Role of Eye-Tracking Technology

Eye tracking is the process of measuring either the point of gaze or the motion of an eye relative to the head. Eye trackers are used in research on the visual system, in psychology, in psycholinguistics, in marketing, as an input device for human-computer interaction, and in product design. Eye-tracking technology has been used on a limited basis in some fields of medicine and nursing, for both training and assessment [21].

For procedural and visual-based tasks, eye tracking holds great promise as a tool for monitoring training progress towards the development of expertise. By recording the direction of a user's gaze and relationship to an area of interest (AOI), eye-tracking technology provides an objective tool for measuring visual patterns. Although gaze patterns captured by eye tracking are not equivalent to cognition, it may bring educators one step closer to making the thought processes of an expert explicit and therefore provide insight into how to guide learners.

This method has been successfully used for proficiency assessment. For example experienced physicians spend more time concentrating on target location while novices split their attention between tracking their tools, the operative site, the sterile field, and the target location [22]. There is recent evidence that novices who were gaze-trained demonstrate target-looking fixation patterns similar to those expressed by experts and gain a performance advantage over trainees left to discover their own strategies for task comple-

tion [23]. This may have interesting implications for the creation of assessment programs, which distinguish skill level through the use of gaze behavior (Fig. 10.7).

10.4 My Teaching Module

In this section I describe my method of teaching epidural as I practice it and have practiced it since the 1980s, including the latest updates I have recently introduced. It does not claim either to be exhaustive or to represent the working model, but I hope that it can be a good starting point for fellow readers who want to undertake or perfect their teaching activity at their institutions.

10.4.1 Anatomy Laboratory

"The real voyage of discovery is not seeing new worlds but changing eyes" (Proust).

Usually trainees have already received a standard front lecture on anatomy and technique during their curriculum. The first module of my teaching method aims to change the trainee's knowledge from a two-dimensional to a three-dimensional vision of the epidural region anatomy. The first step is the assessment of the novice's personal knowledge of what he/she already knows. Students are invited to write down on a sheet the tissues that the needle must pass through to reach the epidural space, both median and paramedian. After that, each student must write on a visual analogue scale how much anxiety this task causes and how satisfied he/she is with the description made. After this first self-awareness of their knowledge, I begin to explain the basics of three-dimensional anatomy using plastic vertebral models that are distributed to each of the students. This "anatomy laboratory" consists of the teacher's explanation with the lumbar vertebral model followed by the construction of an epidural model by learners with various plastic materials representing ligaments. After the construction of the epidural model, more detailed information and comparison with the information contained in the anatomy texts

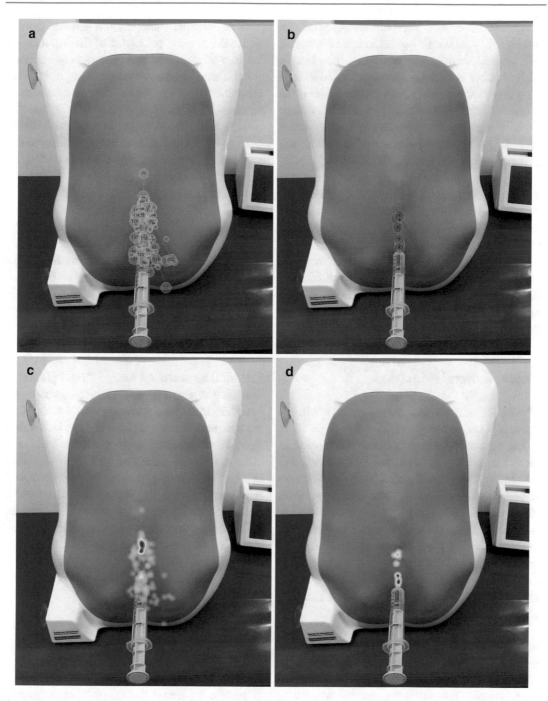

Fig. 10.7 Eye tracking for epidural technique proficiency assessment. Gaze behavior is used to distinguish skill level. Typical novice's (**a**) and expert's (**b**) gaze plots and novice's (**c**) and expert's (**d**) heatmap

and the micro- and macroscopic anatomy of the anatomical structure involved in the lumbar epidural block is provided. Students are then invited to recap, summarize, and describe again the layers that the needle must pass through to reach the epidural space by median and paramedian approach. The typical questions at this stage are as follows: What have you consolidated?

(Confirmation of what I already knew.) What did you learn? What didn't you understand? What do you want to learn more about? (I would like to study it better at home.) Students are also invited to try to draw what they have learned. The most frequent discoveries of my trainees at this stage of their learning are the existence of a supra-interspinous ligament complex and the belonging of these ligaments to the thoracolumbar fascia; the key elements for the success of the block: the vertebral arch and the yellow ligament; the existence of two ligamenta flava and their median hiatus; the function and the real distribution of epidural fat; the dimensions of the ligaments and epidural space; the three-dimensional structure and distribution of the meninges, in particular the disposition of the arachnoid membranes around the spinal roots; and the topographic anatomy of the spinal roots.

10.4.2 General Principles

"Everything must be learned not to exhibit it, but to use it" (Lichtenberg).

In this module I introduce the materials needed to perform an epidural block. Each student has a Touhy needle, a LOR syringe, an epidural catheter, a filter, a connector, a syringe, and a vial of saline. Trainees are encouraged to familiarize themselves with the materials provided, observing their details, connections, and measurements. The teacher will then present the various models of needles and catheters on the market, highlighting the common parts, similarities, and differences.

The second part of this module is the familiarization with the general principles of the loss of resistance technique. The background idea is the following: "You cannot lose what you have not yet acquired." This phase focuses exclusively on the recognition of the increase of resistance (ligamentum flavum) and the loss of resistance (epidural space). The teacher explains the reasons for the use of LOR in the lumbar epidural block, mentioning the existence of other techniques for the thoracic and cervical epidural. Using a Touhy needle, a LOR syringe filled with saline, and a

cube of silicone material, the teacher demonstrates the general principles of the increase and the loss of resistance. A specifically designed video is usually employed at this stage. After the video the trainees perform a practical exercise of increase and loss of resistance with the needle, syringe, and silicone cube. Discussion and clarification with the students on the general principles end this section. Once again, before ending the section the teacher asks the trainees: What have you consolidated? (Confirmation of what you already knew.) What did you learn? What didn't you understand? What do you want to learn more about? (I would like to study it better at home.) How much anxiety did this section cause? How satisfied are you with your learning so far?

10.4.3 Fundamentals with the Epidural Simulator

This section is what I named "The epidural in four steps." Students are in small groups and everyone must try several times. In this phase, the simulator is used exclusively as a task trainer through which the Tuohy needle is passed in order to appreciate and recognize the differences in resistance offered by the fabrics encountered. It is very important to have a simulator which adequately reproduces the different layers the epidural needle must pass to reach the epidural space and for this reason I have modified a commercially available simulator to make it reliable and more similar to human tissues [5] (Fig. 10.8). These are the four basic steps:

1. Recognizing the increase of resistance (ligamentum flavum): If the needle is inserted in the ligamentum flavum, this is confirmed by a slight pressure on the piston: if the piston does not move forward this means that the tip of the needle is sealed by the dense ligamentum flavum. By continuously and steadily but decisively increasing the pressure on the plunger, the needle progresses in the ligamentum against resistance. The trainee must carefully observe that the needle slowly penetrates the tissues while the piston remains stationary.

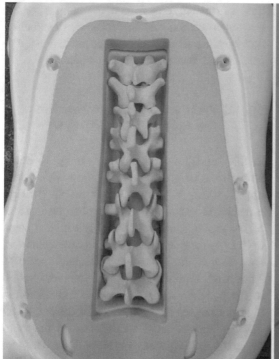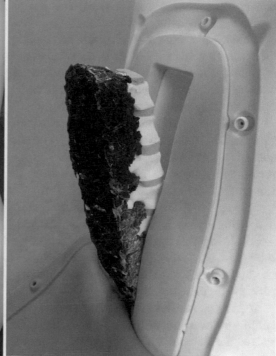

Fig. 10.8 The validated, custom-made epidural simulator, created by modifying the inner structure of a commercially available one, and using some materials of our own design to make it adequately realistic. For detailed information in [5]

2. Recognizing the loss of resistance (epidural space): By pushing progressively and steadily on the piston when the needle is in the ligamentum flavum, as soon as the tip of the needle has reached the epidural space, the piston is suddenly and unequivocally pushed forward and the saline solution is suddenly discharged into the epidural space. At the same time, the progression of the needle stops automatically.
3. Recognizing the false loss of resistance: If the needle is not inserted in the ligamentum flavum, this is confirmed by making a slight pressure on the piston: if the piston moves forward its tip is not in the inextensible, dense ligamentum flavum, but somewhere in the soft tissues, which are easily infiltrated by water.
4. Recognizing the false increase in resistance (bone contact): Resistance may be lost even when the tip of the needle is against a bone (usually the vertebral lamina). However, by increasing the pressure on the plunger contin-

uously and steadily but decisively, the needle does NOT progress into the tissues against resistance.

10.4.4 Teaching by Using Dynamic Pressure Sensing Technology (CompuFlo Trainer®)

I named this section: "See and listen to what you feel."

Students are divided into small groups and everyone must try several times. In this module the epidural simulator is still used exclusively as a task trainer through which the Tuohy needle is passed. The aim is to let trainees appreciate and know how to recognize the differences in resistance offered by the fabrics encountered by having an objective feedback.

For this section I use the CompuFlo Epidural Trainer® which is based on Dynamic Pressure

Sensing® technology (see Chap. 6). This instrument is able to detect pressure changes imperceptible by touch and presents visual and audible feedback allowing the trainee to accurately confirm the location of the needle and consistently discriminate between false and true loss of resistance encountered during the procedure.

After having explained the general principles of operation, the analysis of the graph, and the acoustics of the instrument, the exercises of the previous module are repeated with the help of the CompuFlo Epidural Trainer®.

The epidural Tuohy needle, attached to an anti-reflux valve, is connected to a three-way stopcock, a LOR syringe, and the CompuFlo® tubing extension (Fig. 10.9). The epidural Tuohy needle is slowly advanced with open communication to all three connections.

If at any point in the process there is uncertainty, confusion, or an inconclusive interpretation, the trainee must stop the advancement of the needle and use the instrument to verify the needle position by using the four typical patterns displayed by the CompuFlo Epidural Trainer®: "false increase or decrease of resistance," "bony contact," "needle in the ligamentum flavum," and "needle in the epidural space" (Fig. 10.10). By using the CompuFlo Epidural Trainer® instrument the instructor, who previously depended on the student feedback of tactile feel during the epidural procedure, is, with this instrument, empowered to monitor needle movement on the screen. Procedure documentation is also generated to enhance educational discussion and monitor skill development.

10.4.5 Problem Setting: Introducing the Epidural Checklist

In this educational module it is tough to know how to reduce the complexity of the epidural technique. At this stage the teacher should perform a masterful execution of the technique in front of the students, illustrating all the logical steps of the performance of the epidural technique, according to the institutional standard checklist, from hand scrubbing to epidural catheter fixation to the patient's skin. The teacher illustrates the algorithm of the epidural checklist (poster, slide) and explains in detail all the steps of the technique by dividing them into several blocks.

After careful observation, the trainees are invited to imagine the steps and write them down on a piece of paper (mentalization procedure) highlighting areas for improvement in their personal training experience. It may be useful at this stage to use individual games to reinforce the epidural checklist learning, such as making a puzzle in which pieces depict the epidural checklist in a sequential and chronological way.

Fig. 10.9 The connections between the epidural needle, the LOR syringe, and the CompuFlo Epidural Trainer® used for teaching purposes

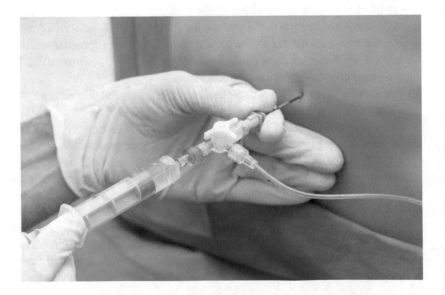

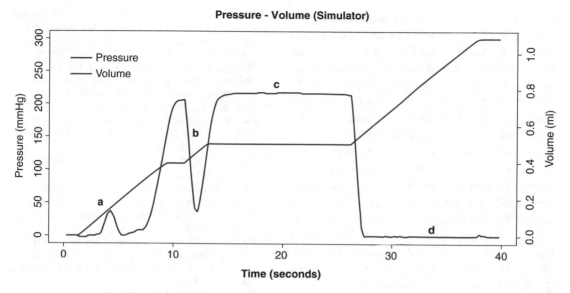

Fig. 10.10 Typical pressure-volume infused curve during identification of the epidural procedure with the simulator and the CompuFlo Epidural Trainer®: (a) subcutaneous tissues and/or supraspinous ligament; (b) false loss of resistance; (c) ligamentum flavum; (d) epidural space

10.4.6 "Hands-On" Technique Using the Epidural Simulator

"No one can understand something well and make it their own when they have learned it from another, compared to when they have learned it on their own" (Descartes).

At this stage the trainee is ready to perform the various steps of the technique on the epidural simulator, prepared ad hoc so as to reproduce and re-propose the development of the real technique (sterile cloths, gloves, hat and mask, preparation of the trolley, local anesthesia, etc.). Performance is eventually evaluated with checklists and the Global Assessment Rate both by the students (self-assessment) and by an independent instructor.

10.4.7 Epidural Block as in the Real World: High-Fidelity Simulation

"True truths are those that can be invented" (Kraus).

At this stage the execution of the technique is performed in the high-fidelity simulation room in a realistic environment reproducing the deliv-ery room and/or the operating room, by using scenarios with actors (patient, nurse, colleague) and/or a high-fidelity manikin. The trainee's performance evaluation is made by debriefing with the help of checklists and the Global Assessment Rate (Fig. 10.3).

10.4.8 Training on the Patient

"We're not doing anything right until we stop thinking about how to do it" (Hazlitt).

According to local institutional rotation and policy, this part of the training is carried out in the operating and/or labor and delivery rooms. The instructor performs the technique in front of the trainee in a masterful way. On this occasion, materials, procedures, and general principles are reviewed together with the trainee. Basically, this stage of teaching has four phases. In the first phase the teacher performs the technique and the pupil, with sterile gloves, puts his/her hands exactly on those of the tutor, who will communicate aloud all the passages of the needle in the tissues associating the tactile sensations and anatomical structures crossed. In my experience the first 5–10 epidurals should be performed in this way. In the second phase, the pupil performs the technique and the teacher, with sterile gloves, puts his/her hands exactly on those of the pupil, who will communicate aloud all the passages of the needle in the tissues, attempting to correlate tactile sensations and anatomical structures crossed. The teacher confirms the tactile sensations of the pupil at each step. Ten additional epidurals should be performed in this way. In the third phase the pupil performs the technique completely alone, but the teacher is next to him/her. Observation and intervention occur only if required and necessary. During the fourth stage the trainee performs the technique completely alone. The teacher is not in the same room but is readily available on request. The number of epidurals necessary for the transition from phase one to phase four may vary according to the teacher's judgement, the pupil's performance, and the technical difficulties that occurred during the training. For a better understanding of the evolution of the trainee during this period of learning the use of CUSUM curves may be beneficial for both trainee and teacher.

References

1. Birnbach DJ, Santos AC, Bourlier RA, et al. The effectiveness of video technology as an adjunct to teach and evaluate epidural anesthesia performance skills. Anesthesiology. 2002;96:5–9.
2. Tien JC, Lim MJ, Leong WL, et al. Nine-year audit of post-dural puncture headache in a tertiary obstetric hospital in Singapore. Int J Obstet Anesth. 2016;28:34–8.
3. Vaugham N, Dubey VN, Wee MYK, et al. Advanced epidural simulator with 3D flexible spine and haptic Interface. J Med Devices. 2014;6:017524.
4. Ghelber O, Gebhard R, Katz J, et al. The CompuFlo® helps inexperienced operators identify the epidural space in a simulator model. EJA. 2006;23:242.
5. Capogna G, Coccoluto A, Capogna E, et al. Objective evaluation of a new epidural simulator by the CompuFlo® epidural instrument. Anesthesiol Res Pract. 2018;2018:4710263.
6. Capogna E, Coccoluto A, Gibiino G, et al. CompuFlo® assisted training vs conventional training for the identification of the ligamentum flavum with an epidural simulator: a brief report. Anesthesiol Res Pract. 2019;2019:3804743.
7. Friedman Z, Katznelson R, Devito I, et al. Objective assessment of manual skills and proficiency in performing epidural anesthesia-video-assisted validation. Reg Anesth Pain Med. 2006;31:304–10.
8. Ringsted C, Ostergaard D, Scherpbier A. Embracing the new paradigm of assessment in residency training: an assessment programme for first-year residency training in anesthesiology. Med Teach. 2003;25:54–62.
9. Sivarajan M, Miller E, Hardy C, et al. Objective evaluation of clinical performance and correlation with knowledge. Anesth Analg. 1984;63:603–7.
10. McKinley RK, Strand J, Ward L, et al. Checklists for assessment and certification of clinical procedural skills omit essential competencies: a systematic review. Med Educ. 2008;42:338–49.
11. Wright TP. Factors affecting the cost of airplanes. J Aeronaut Sci. 1936;3:122–8.
12. Kopacz DJ, Neal JM, Pollock JE. The regional anesthesia 'learning curve'. What is the minimum number of epidural and spinal blocks to reach consistency? Reg Anesth. 1996;21:182–90.
13. Starkie T, Drake EJ. Assessment of procedural skills training and performance in anesthesia using cumulative sum analysis (cusum). Can J Anaesth. 2013;60:1228–39.
14. Drake EJ, Coghill J, Sneyd JR. Defining competence in obstetric epidural anaesthesia for inexperienced trainees. BJA. 2015;114:951–571.
15. Ahlberg G, Enochsson L, Gallagher AG, et al. Proficiency-based virtual reality training significantly reduces the error rate for residents during their first 10 laparoscopic cholecystectomies. Am J Surg. 2007;193:797–804.
16. Zivkovic N, van Samkar G, Hermanns H, et al. Face and construct validity of TU-Delft epidural simulator and the value of real-time visualization. Reg Anesth Pain Med. 2019. pii: rapm-2018-100161. https://doi.org/10.1136/rapm-2018-100161. [Epub ahead of print].
17. Friedman Z, Siddiqui N, Katznelson R, et al. Clinical impact of epidural Anesthesia simulation on short- and long-term learning curve: high- versus low-fidelity model training. Reg Anesth Pain Med. 2009;34:229–32.
18. Beed P, Hawkins M, Roller C. Moving learners towards independence: the power of scaffolded instruction. Read Teach. 1991;44:648–55.
19. Reznick R, Regehr G, MacRae H, et al. Testing technical skill via an innovative 'bench station' examination. Am J Surg. 1997;173:226–30.
20. Martin JA, Regehr G, Reznick R, et al. Objective structured assessment of technical skill (OSATS) for surgical residents. Br J Surg. 1997;84:273–8.
21. Tien T, Pucher PH, Sodergren MH, et al. Eye tracking for skills assessment and training: a systematic review. J Surg Res. 2014;191:169–78.
22. Khan RS, Tien G, Atkins MS, et al. Analysis of eye gaze: do novice surgeons look at the same location as expert surgeons during a laparoscopic operation? Surg Endosc Other Interv Tech. 2012;26:3536–40.
23. Vine SJ, Masters RS, McGrath JS, et al. Cheating experience: guiding novices to adopt the gaze strategies of experts expedites the learning of technical laparoscopic skills. Surgery. 2012;152:32–40.

The Words of the Masters

In this chapter the original words of our masters are reported, how they have described the epidural technique and how they performed it. What they have described in the past is still invaluable today, despite the technical advances in the materials and the development of new technologies.

11.1 Achille M. Dogliotti (1897–1966)

This is the very first description Dogliotti made during the departmental meeting of April 18th, 1931, when he reported his very initial experience on 18 patients who underwent lumbar epidural anesthesia [1]: "The technique of injection, though it may seem very delicate, is actually usually easy if you pay attention to the following facts. Everyone who has some experience in spinal puncture knows that some uniform fibrous resistance is encountered during the progression of the needle in the thickness of the interspinous and intervertebral ligament. If during this first time we remove the stylet and try to inject some liquid, we find a strong resistance. Continuing the advancement of the needle, the hand, and often also the eye of the operator, feels a first click, almost as if suddenly a good part of the previous resistance to the progress of the needle was missing. If the advance of the needle has been slow and cautious, you can immediately stop the needle as soon as you feel this click. If at this point we remove the stylet, nothing comes out. If we inject liquid this enters with extreme ease, does not meet any resistance, we almost have the impression of putting it in a vacuum."

One year later he reported his final, and now well-proven, loss-of-resistance technique at the 12th Annual Congress of Anesthesiologists, in New York City in October 1932 [2]: "When the needle has penetrated the ligamentum interspinous for a certain distance and before it has gone through the ligamenta subflava into the spinal canal one removes the trocar and attaches a syringe filled with physiological saline. When an attempt is made to inject this fluid a very great resistance is met with since the interspinous ligamentum and the ligamenta subflava are so dense. If they can be injected at all, it will be only after the employment of considerable force. This resistance is most certain evidence that the needle is still in the posterior fibers of these tissues. The following maneuvers are then carried out: the syringe is held in one hand the thumb of which applies a continued and uniform pressure to the piston (Fig. 1.6). The other hand slowly advances the needle into the tissues and when it has traversed a few millimeters the hand which is holding it will suddenly note a diminution in the resistance to its passage which has previously been due to the tissues of the ligamenta subflava. At the same instant the injection fluid enters freely. This is certain, practical and unequivocal evidence that the point of the needle has pierced

G. Capogna, *Epidural Technique In Obstetric Anesthesia*, https://doi.org/10.1007/978-3-030-45332-9_11

the ligamenta subflava and is in the peridural space which offers no resistance to the flow of the injected fluid. As soon as this position has been recognized the needle should be left in the position which it now occupies for its point is in the peridural space; any attempt to advance it farther would entail the risk of penetrating the dura."

11.2   John J. Bonica (1917–1994)

This is the original description Bonica made in the 1950s in his masterpiece *Management of Pain* [3]: "Just before the point of the needle has engaged the ligamentum flavum, the stylet is removed, and an attempt is made to inject saline with a 5 cc. Luer lock syringe. If the bevel of the needle is within the compact ligamentum flavum this attempt will meet with considerable resistance, whereas if the bevel is still in the loose interspinous ligament the resistance will be of only moderate degree. With a little practice, vari-

ous degrees of resistance, as the needle passes through the various structures, become better appreciated and are more easily discernible. While the thumb of the right hand exerts constant, unremitting, steady pressure on the plunger of the syringe, the shaft of the needle is grasped between the thumb and forefinger of the left hand and very slowly advanced (Fig. 11.1). The left hand should rest on the back of the patient as so to steady the needle and better regulate the pressure that is exerted against it. In this manner the needle is very slowly and gently pushed through the ligamentum flavum until it enters the peridural space. As soon as the bevel begins to enter this space, there is a sudden lack of resistance, and the liquid, which up to this point had encountered great resistance, now escapes very rapidly and freely, whereupon the needle is arrested."

And this is the same description 10 years later [4]: "As soon as the needle point reaches the supraspinous ligament, greater resistance is encountered because of the nature of the bevel

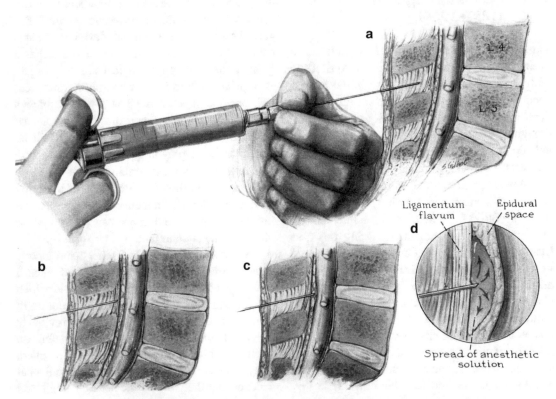

Fig. 11.1 Bonica's technique: (**a**) advance of the needle with left hand while constant unremitting pressure is being exerted on the plunger of the syringe. (**b**) needle point in the ligamentum flavum, which offers great resis-

tance. (**c**) entrance of point of needle into epidural space is discerned by sudden lack of resistance to the injection of the saline. (**d**) diffusion of the solution throughout the epidural space and the density of the ligament. The needle is then advanced 2.5–3 cm through the loose interspinous ligament which offers less resistance. When the needle engages the ligamentum flavum, more resistance is encountered: the stylet is removed and the 10 mL. Luer-Lock control syringe filled with saline is carefully adapted to the needle (use of air, because of its compressibility, decreases the sensitivity to pressure changes as resistance is met). If the operator is right-handed, it is easier to manage the syringe with the right hand, while the needle is grasped firmly between the thumb and the index finger of the left hand and the other fingers and the back of left hand rest against the patient's back. An attempt is then made to inject the saline. If the point of the needle is still in the interspinous ligament, only moderate resistance to the injection is encountered, but if it is in the tough, dense ligamentum flavum, attempts to inject are met with considerable resistance. The point of the needle must be advanced very slowly, through the ligamentum flavum, while the thumb of the right hand exerts *constant, unremitting pressure* on the plunger of the syringe. Some physicians prefer to advance the needle intermittently 1–2 mm. and then to stop and apply pressure on the plunger; the maneuver is repeated several times until the point of the needle enters the space. The importance of moving the needle through the ligamentum flavum *very slowly* cannot be overemphasized; 20–30 s should be allowed to advance the needle through the 3–5 mm thickness of the ligament.

As soon as the bevel of the needle enters the peridural space there is a sudden lack of resistance and the liquid, which to this point has encountered obstruction, now escapes rapidly and freely. *The advance of the needle is stopped instantly on entering the space* and the solution is discharged. When the bevel of the needle is wholly within the peridural space, it is possible to inject saline with little or no resistance: the feeling is the same as injecting fluid into the subarachnoid space. If the operator experiences the sudden marked decrease in resistance, indicating passage of the point of the needle through the ligament, but still feels that the injection is not free or there is reflux of the fluid, the point of

the needle is either not entirely within the epidural space or contains a particle of tissue, which was 'punched out' by the bevel. To eliminate these possibilities, the stylet is replaced into the needle, and the needle *slowly* advanced 2–3 mm and injection again attempted. If resistance is still encountered or there is still reflux, the needle has missed its target and should be withdrawn and another attempt made" (Fig. 11.2).

11.3   Daniel C. Moore (1918–2015)

In the years after World War II, questions were raised about the safety and utility of regional blockade. Daniel C. Moore emerged as an enthusiastic advocate of regional techniques, effectively leading a renaissance of regional anesthesia interest through his textbook, teaching, and research. This is his description [5]: "If the anesthesiologist is right-handed, the index finger and the thumb of the right hand grasp the hub of the needle while the other fingers and back of the hand rest firmly against the patient's back. Firm, continuous pressure is exerted against the plunger of the syringe with the left hand (Fig. 11.3). If the needle lies within the substance of the anterior intraspinous ligament or the ligamentum flavum, it is very difficult to force any of the saline from the syringe. The index finger and thumb of the right hand now very slowly advance the needle while constant, unremitting, pressure is kept on the plunger of the syringe with the left hand. The moment the bevel of the needle enters the epidural space, the contents of the syringe will be rapidly discharged if constant, unremitting, pressure on the plunger has been exerted. The forward advancement of the needle is immediately stopped, and if this advancement has been very slow and cautious, the bevel of the needle will lie in the epidural space."

11.4   P. R. Bromage (1920–2013)

This is the exhaustive description of the position of the operator's hands suggested by Bromage in his popular textbook [6]: "A firm, braced grip

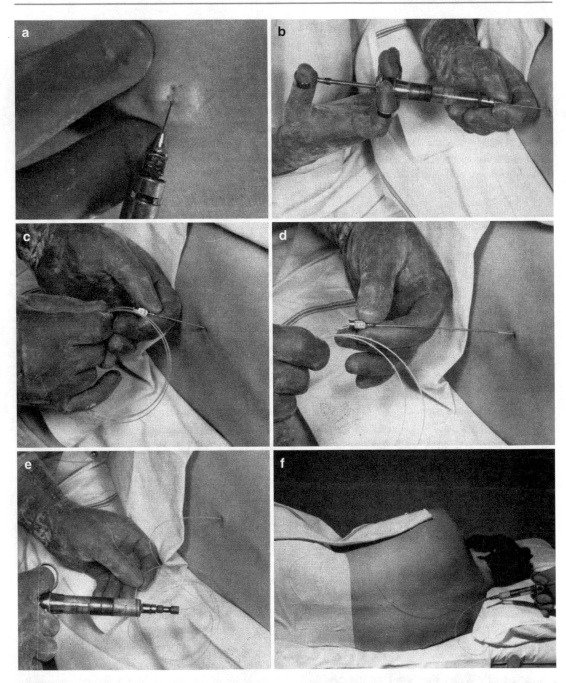

Fig. 11.2 Bonica's technique, paramedian approach. (**a**) formation of intracutaneous wheal just lateral to lower portion of spinous process of third lumbar vertebra. (**b**) advance of the needle. (**c**) introduction of the catheter. (**d**) withdrawal of the needle over the tubing. (**e**) injection of the test dose. (**f**) catheter is imobilized with adhesive tape: note the large circle made by the catheter to decrease risk of kinking at its point of exit from the skin

on the needle and a slow, controlled advance are among the most essential conditions for the technique … The grip on the needle is all-important and is designed to reduce the natural compliance and elasticity in the operator's hand to a mini-mum, so that the needle is advanced steadily and evenly as if by a machine under micrometric control. The needle is grasped at the junction of the hub and shaft so that the grip exerts a three-point fixation (Fig. 11.4). The needle is gripped

Fig. 11.3 Moore's technique. (**a**) needle rests in interspinous ligament. (**b**) needle rests in epidural space

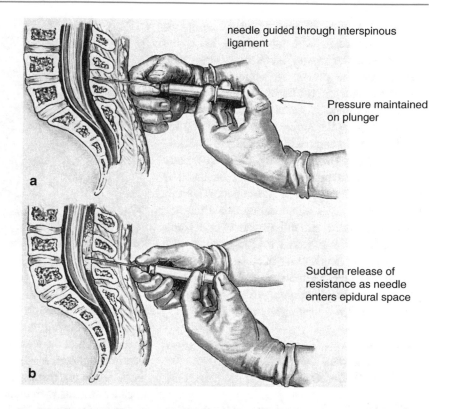

needle guided through interspinous ligament

Pressure maintained on plunger

Sudden release of resistance as needle enters epidural space

Fig. 11.4 Bromage's technique

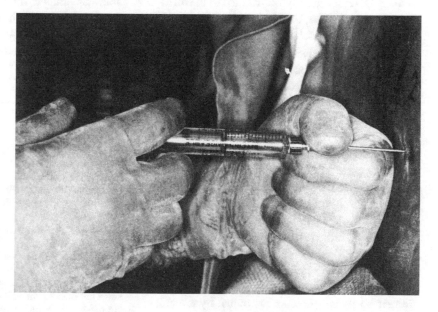

between the thumb on top and the proximal and distal phalanges of the crooked forefinger below. The hand is supinated, with the wrist partially flexed and the back of the carpus braced against the patient's back. Forward motion is imparted to the needle by a gradual extension of the wrist, and the carpus and metacarpus roll in toward the back like an eccentric cam driving a piston. The hand must be rock-steady to supply a gradual, controlled forward movement to the needle, as well as an instantaneous braking force as soon as the epidural space is entered. The forward movement should be gradual and continuous, never intermittent. The other hand holds the syringe, and the thumb exerts continuous firm pressure on the plunger, sensing the different resistances encountered during the advance of the needle. This hand is almost entirely concerned with supporting the syringe and interpreting the significance of changes in resistance to injection as the needle advances; the slight forward motion that it imparts to the needle is counterbalanced by the other hand braced against the patient's back. A 5-mL syringe is small enough to allow the backs of the fourth and fifth fingers of both hands to remain in contact and braced against each other. The two hands move in concert like a slow exercise in isometric contraction. *Never advance the needle without simultaneous pressure on the plunger to tell you where you are.*"

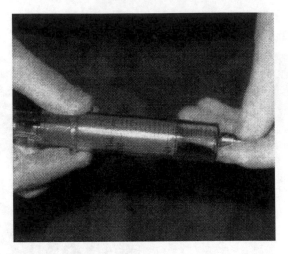

Fig. 11.5 Doughty's technique

11.5   Andrew Doughty (1916–2013)

Andrew Doughty greatly contributed to the diffusion of epidural labor analgesia in the UK. In this letter [7] he explains the technical variant he popularized in the 1960s–1970s: "With the operator standing side-on to the patient, the epidural needle is pushed into the back by the pressure of the right thumb, index and middle fingers gripping the rim of the proximal end of a 20 mL syringe (Fig. 11.5). The *right* hand is thus responsible for appreciating the resistance of the ligamentum flavum. The controlling or braking force is applied in an opposite direction by the grip of the fingers and thumb of the *left* hand on the hub of the needle, the knuckles resting against the patient's back. The 'indicator equipment' responsible for demonstrating the entry of the needle point into the epidural space is a scrupulously clean all-glass 20 mL syringe with a smooth-running plunger on which pressure is applied by the ball of the index finger or the palm of the right hand during the advance of the Tuohy needle: thus the considerable force which may be required to pro-

pel the needle through the ligamentum flavum is separated from the small and delicate pressure needed to elicit the loss of resistance to injection. I do not expect to make converts to my technique from among experienced operators achieving excellent results with methods to which they have become accustomed, but I strongly recommend it as one that I have taught to beginners for many years and with which they have quickly acquired confidence; for them I have found it *almost* 'dural puncture proof!'"

References

1. Dogliotti AM. Un promettente metodo di anestesia tronculare in studio: la rachianestesia peridurale segmentaria. Bollettino della Società Piemontese di Chirurgia. 1931;I:385–99.
2. Dogliotti AM. Trattato di Anestesia. Torino: UTET; 1946.
3. Bonica JJ. The management of pain. Philadelphia: Lea & Febiger; 1953.
4. Moore DC. Regional block. Springfield: CC Thomas; 1953.
5. Bonica JJ. Principles and practice of obstetric analgesia & anesthesia. Philadelphia: FA Davies Co.; 1967.
6. Bromage PR. Epidural analgesia. Philadelphia: WB Saunders Co.; 1978.
7. Doughty A. Self arresting epidural introducer. Anaesthesia. 1982;37:470.

Printed in the United States
by Baker & Taylor Publisher Services